BEAUTY
BY
DESIGN
a complete look at

COSMETIC
SURGERY

BEAUTY
BY
DESIGN
a complete look at

COSMETIC
SURGERY

Kurt J. Wagner, M.D.
and
Gerald Imber, M.D.

McGraw-Hill Book Company

New York   St. Louis   San Francisco

Toronto   Düsseldorf   Mexico

To Eileen Imber and Kathie Wagner for their unflagging enthusiasm and encouragement through the dark moments of this project. Special thanks to Peter Cardozo and Robert Hirsch for professional guidance and friendship which added greatly to the book.

GI and KJW

Library of Congress Cataloging in Publication Data

Wagner, Kurt
  Beauty by design.
  1. Surgery, Plastic. I. Imber, Gerald, joint
author. II. Title.
RD119.W32   617'.95   78-10818
ISBN 0-07-067671-2

CONTENTS

INTRODUCTION

IS COSMETIC SURGERY FOR YOU?

In today's world this is a question worth considering.
Beauty is such a desirable characteristic.
It seems to be a passport to the life we want to live.
We're all interested in looking well. If we feel we are aging, if the face reflected in the mirror is less perfect than we would like, then certainly it is not surprising that we daydream about improving the way we look.

We all want to look our best. Today we are free to make this statement in word and deed, without guilt. Physical fitness has become a way of life. The beauty and fashion industries are booming. Millions of people are seeking self-improvement through diet, sports and dress. In short, self-awareness has come out of the closet. Yet all of these measures may not prove quite enough to create the beautiful sense of self that so many of us wish to hold out to the world. Hence the question, "Is cosmetic surgery for you"?

AGAIN THE QUESTION: IS COSMETIC SURGERY FOR YOU?

Cosmetic surgery is no longer reserved for the rich and famous, the millionaire socialites, and TV and movie stars. Housewives and career women, businessmen and professionals, too, are aware of how cosmetic surgery may reshape faces and bodies, enhance self-image, open new life possibilities, and prevent the door from shutting out youth prematurely. In this book we, as two experienced plastic surgeons, endeavor to anticipate all your questions and to answer them as fully, as fairly, as objectively as can be done without a personal interview.

Over the past few years cosmetic surgery has received a great deal of attention in the media. Newspaper and magazine articles, radio and television programs, have all played a role in the information explosion. Unfortunately, these articles and programs fail to give a balanced picture and tell the whole story. They tend to distort, to tilt opinion too strongly one way or the other. Either they are pro cosmetic surgery: it's magic; it can do no wrong. Or, they're so adamantly against this new science as to deny it any virtue. The truth is, cosmetic surgery can offer new vistas for self-improvement. It can change lives and open the door to a better existence. Yet it is not miraculous. It is a science in the hands of human practitioners and there can be problems. As a rule, the results produced by cosmetic surgery far outweigh any difficulties. The overwhelming percentage of patients become loyal advocates of self-improvement through cosmetic surgery.

The purpose of this book is to guide you to a fuller understanding of cosmetic surgery and to help you decide for yourself whether or not it is for you. As surgeons, we believe that you as a consumer of medical care need to know, and deserve to know, about all the possibilities and pitfalls you face. This book will serve you as a consumers' guide to the world of cosmetic surgery. For each type of surgery, we will discuss the sort of patient who would most benefit, the treatment before and after, the likely results, and the most common complications. Like most surgeons we heartily subscribe to the patient's right to know. We want our patients to enjoy a full and clear knowledge of the surgery to be performed. This makes the entire experience as positive and rewarding as it should be.

The so-called "magic" of cosmetic surgery is really the result of a careful, thoughtful, balanced plan for esthetic improvement. The specialist is highly trained in manipulating anatomy and nature to the patient's advantage. If there is some minor magic, you will soon have a clearer understanding of how it is performed. To help, we have drawn freely from our own experience and extensive interviews with our patients. This enables us to see the picture from your point of view. We think we know what is on your mind when we discuss cosmetic surgery. By now we are aware of the truths, half-truths, and myths you have been asked to believe. Hopefully, this book will set things straight; certainly, it was written with you in mind.

In these pages you will find issues on which not all cosmetic surgeons agree. However, most of these will be small points that will usually be lost in a sea of general agreement. It is not our intention to conflict with or criticize the methods or ideas of other physicians. We are not the last word, nor are we convinced that the last word exists. In medicine results are often obtained by widely different means. If you read this book for background information before cosmetic surgery, you will possibly find a few points where we differ from the opinions and instructions of the surgeon you have chosen. The solution to this dilemma is clear. The best source of information for you is *your* surgeon. It is not our desire to intrude on this all-important professional relationship. Our purpose is to provide an overview and guidance in understanding the value and the limits of cosmetic surgery.

CHAPTER 1

WHAT TO EXPECT
FROM A FACE LIFT

The familiar term *face lift* is more fully descriptive and a great deal easier to understand than more technical words sometimes used in medical circles to discuss this common procedure. The terms *rhytidectomy*, which means excision of wrinkles, *rhytidoplasty*, which means molding of wrinkles, and *meloplasty*, which means something like molding of the face, do little to describe the surgery and a great deal to confound communication. Although some surgeons may consider the expression *face lift* beneath their dignity, we feel that it is a good one because it is universally understood by patients and the public at large. It is therefore the term we shall use throughout this book.

The only problem with the phrase *face lift* may be that it encourages unrealistic expectations in some patients. The expression is now so much a part of our language that it is difficult to determine whether it was first devised to describe the surgical procedure, or applied to the procedure after having been accepted in other contexts. In either case, we know that when someone says that a store or other building is "having its face lifted," we are meant to understand that its old face is being replaced with a new one. Unfortunately, this is not the case in surgical face lifting. To a plastic surgeon, performing a face lift is more like giving the patient back his or her more youthful face.

If you are thinking of a face lift, you can realistically expect it to do a great deal to remove any hanging skin and wrinkles you may have, and generally to erase the ravages of time upon the facial skin. Even the most successful surgical face lift, however, can only turn back the clock. Although you may appear much as you did five, ten or fifteen years ago, before loose skin and wrinkles may have given you an older and more tired appearance, you will still be the same person. If you were unhappy with your facial appearance ten years ago, having a face lift will not, by itself, be the complete answer for you.

A face lift, however, is far from being the only kind of surgery that can produce improvement. Other procedures often performed with the face lift can not only help to remove signs of aging but can change the patient's facial features for the better. Many surgeons routinely smooth out eyelid wrinkles, remove loose "turkey gobbler" skin under the chin, change the size and shape of the nose, enlarge the chin, augment the cheekbones, or even pin back the ears, along with a face lift, if they and the patient feel that any of these procedures will improve the overall result. If you think you would benefit from one or more of these other changes, the time to let your surgeon know about it is at your consultation.

Even if you enjoyed the way your face looked ten years ago, you may still want to consider one or more of these additional procedures. As the skin begins to droop, a number of other changes occur as well. The skin beneath the jaw begins to hang, the tip of the nose begins to point increasingly downward. In general, gravity is less effectively opposed. Although not everyone needs such changes, a straight nose, strong chin and reduced "turkey neck," in addition to your face lift, should greatly improve the outcome. Don't be surprised, therefore, if your surgeon brings up one or more of these ideas for your consideration.

A preliminary consultation with a plastic surgeon is no time to be self-conscious or reserved. This is your best opportunity to discuss openly and frankly what you don't like about your appearance, and the changes you would like to see. Don't be shy about listing them. There is nothing whatever wrong in wanting to look your best, and there are no Brownie points for those who choose to look old and tired. The choice, and the right to choose, are yours alone. However, not every surgical procedure is proper for every individual. This is particularly true in the case of the face lift.

WHY DOES FACIAL SKIN SAG?

In the diagram below, the face has been arbitrarily divided into three sections: the upper or temporal area, the middle section, and the lower or cervical (neck) area. In life, of course, each of these sections flows into the next and it is impossible to delineate the boundaries exactly. However, a rough three-way division is useful because the facial changes of aging often affect these

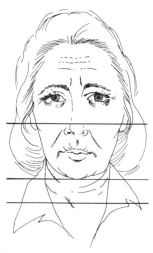

areas selectively, and corrective procedures are aimed at them individually.

In early adult life, numerous biochemical changes take place within the skin. Among these are changes affecting those important components of the dermis, or deep layer, of the skin which are called elastic fibers. It is these fibers which allow skin to stretch, then return to its shape each time the elbow is bent or the face distorted in a grimace. Integrity of the elastic fibers is also responsible, in large part, for the ability of the skin to shrink following weight loss. Although a young person may lose a great deal of weight and still have tight, youthful skin, a middle-aged individual who loses 50 pounds is generally left with loose-hanging skin. Elastic and other connective tissue fibers, which once bound the skin tenaciously to the muscles and other anatomical structures beneath and allowed it to spring back after being stretched, can no longer perform their task. Aging skin thus has less resilience and can no longer bounce back against the pull of gravity. Elastic fiber content in the skin varies considerably among normal individuals and with age.

Passage of time also brings marked diminution in the blood flow within the small vessels which nourish the skin. The decrease is gradual in most cases, but is accentuated by activities such as cigarette smoking. This decrease in blood flow results in changes in the quality of the skin and its fat padding which are manifested as a loss of tone. It also produces changes in the quality of the skin as a whole.

The processes of aging and loss of elasticity are also hastened by prolonged and intensive exposure to the sun. Excessive use of alcohol, poor nutrition, and lack of sleep and exercise also aid in the assault on the skin. Soon the downward pull of gravity cannot be effectively overcome by natural forces. At this point, whether there is just a little loosening or a general deterioration, no amount of diet or exercise will help. These unfortunate changes can be reversed only by the surgical face lift.

It should be made clear that the elasticity and general health of the skin are in no way improved by undergoing such surgery. What is taking place is simply removal of a portion of the stretched-out skin and redraping of the remaining skin so as to make the loss of elasticity less noticeable. The skill of the surgeon is thus directed at reducing, tightening, and smoothing the skin, and generally at helping to overcome the effects of life style, years, and gravity, upon the face.

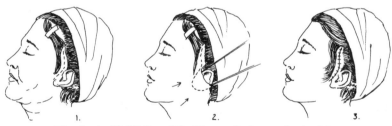

The basic "full" face lift. Figure 1 shows the incision.
Figure 2 the direction of lift. Figure 3 the result. No hair is shaved.

THE TEMPORAL AREA

The temporal or upper face is the area between the hairlines on the sides of the face and from the hairline on the forehead down to the skin below the cheekbones. This is a portion of the face in which early change is often noted. Such a change is especially significant among photographic models whose livelihood depends in large part on a wide-awake, youthful appearance, and in whom even the first signs of aging and sagging are unacceptable. The temporal face lift deals with over-hanging, drooping eyebrows, excessively deep wrinkling of the forehead and loss of high, youthful cheeks.

In the temporal lift operation, the incision begins about midway in front of the ear and is carried, in a C-shaped curve within the hairline, up to an area above the eye-brow. The tissues are carefully lifted and replaced in po-sitions they formerly occupied, the excess skin is surgically excised, and the wounds are carefully closed. The over-whelming majority of the surgical scar is invisible within the hair. This operation lifts the upper portion of the face. It yields the most dramatic results in individuals with strong cheekbones and thin faces, but all patients with aging changes in this area benefit by varying degrees.

THE MIDDLE AREA

The middle area of the face includes some of the ground covered by the temporal lift, plus the entire cheek to the level of the mandible (jawbone). The operation dealing with this is designed to combat heaviness and drooping of the cheek, folding of the cheek in what is called the nasolabial line between the nose and the corner of the mouth, and development of jowls. The incision is an ex-tended version of the one described for the temporal lift. It moves around or barely inside the front of the ear, under the earlobe, into the crease behind the ear and back into the hairline. This procedure eliminates most of the jowls, yielding a sleek, clean jaw line, and deals effectively with descent of the cheeks, reducing the heaviness of the nasolabial fold.

A face lift does not eliminate the nasolabial fold, nor can it eliminate the nasolabial line. The reason for this is physical. The pulling action of the face lift is most effective when the skin is draped over a prominent bone such as the cheekbone or jaw. The cheek and nasolabial areas, however, consist of a mass of muscle covered on the inside of the mouth by mucosa and on the outside by skin, with no firm structural elements underneath. Because this area is farther from a structural bone than any other dealt with in the face lift, it is less dramatically changed than we would like it to be.

THE NECK AREA

In the cervical area, we see jowls hanging beneath the jaw line, general crepiness of the skin, and often large amounts of loose, hanging skin about the neck. The incisions used in middle face surgery may also be employed here. In most cases, contrary to popular misconception, the best results in this area result from a full face lift and not from a direct "attack" on the neck problems. The full face lift provides a well-camouflaged incision, and the additional upward lift of facial tissues gives a more pleasant overall result.

Division of the face lift into separate areas is artificial. In most cases, aging is noted throughout the face and neck, and the finest results are obtained with a complete face lift. It is a fair generalization that less than a complete face lift will give a less than complete result. Although in exceptional cases problem areas can be dealt with separately, a full face lift usually is indicated for best results.

Often, however, specific "neck problems" are the reason for seeing the plastic surgeon, and the deformities may be profound. This area ages early and disturbingly, and a clean jaw line and neck can give way to wrinkles, prominent vertical bands, and a "turkey gobbler" look within a few years.

In some cases, the cause of a neck problem is individual anatomy. In most profiles, a clear, sharp angle is formed by the jaw and neck. When the hyoid bone is positioned low on the neck, or when there is an abnormal amount of fatty tissue below the jaw, a less sharp angle is formed and the individual therefore appears to have double chins or no chin at all. Here, a face lift is of benefit. The primary objective is to create the illusion of a graceful neck. This is done by masking unsightly anatomical characteristics and eliminating signs of aging. Through a small incision beneath the chin the excess fat of the neck is removed. Through the same incision, a chin implant may be inserted to strengthen the projection of the jaw and produce what is a more attractive angle between the neck and jaw line. The face lift, with particular attention to the neck area, is the basic ingredient of this surgery if excess or aging skin of the neck is to be smoothed and recontoured. Despite the actual surgical improvement and the optical illusion created, absolute correction of the problem is unlikely. The patient must be aware of this prior to surgery, and must be realistic in her expectations.

The "turkey gobbler" appearance so common in middle-aged men is often accentuated by weight loss and the consequent transition from double chin to empty-hanging neck skin. Here, the best results are obtained with a full face lift and an additional incision beneath the chin. The neck incision may be T-shaped in some cases, but it is usually in the shape of one or two Z's. This serves the dual purpose of allowing greater skin removal and decreasing the chances of a foreshortened, unsightly scar. This portion of the procedure is sometimes repeated several months later in order to remove a maximal amount of hanging skin. Many surgeons believe neck skin hanging over a shirt collar or turtleneck is the single factor which most often makes a man seek face and neck lift surgery.

Women most often note general crepiness of the neck skin, and two persistent and unsightly vertical bands beneath the chin which detract from the spare, graceful look that is so pleasant about the neck. These bands are caused by stretching or displacement of the leading edge of a superficial muscle of the neck called the platysma. Many operations have been devised to deal with this problem. They are quite successful, though results are not universally perfect. Here, too, a second incision beneath the chin is often required. This heals with little visible scarring and is a useful adjunct to a face lift. A small enlargement of the chin may add to the grace of the final outcome.

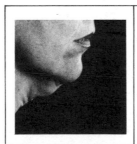 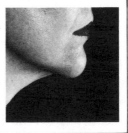

Before: Excess skin beneath jaw.   After neck lift and chin augmentation.

CHAPTER 2

YOUR FACE LIFT: WHAT HAPPENS BEFORE, DURING AND AFTER

"Tell me, Doctor, exactly what should I expect before, during and after the face lift operation?"

This, in one form or another, is a request that we plastic surgeons are receiving constantly—and very understandably—from our patients. In trying to respond to it here, we shall undoubtedly be presenting a picture of our own office routines and procedures rather than those of other surgeons. Obviously, the methods and routines used by others will differ, at least in some respects, and we do not intend to suggest that our own approaches are the only correct ones or to encourage comparisons. Nevertheless, the purpose here is to give you a picture of what is usually involved in a face lift, before, during and after the surgery.

BEFORE THE OPERATION

During the first visit you make to your plastic surgeon, he will undoubtedly ask why you are considering this surgery. He will be hoping that you are a realistic patient who appreciates the possibility of improvement through plastic surgery, but at the same time accepts the limitations and realities of the situation. It is helpful for him to understand your motivation in seeking a face lift. This consultation is an opportunity for doctor and patient to get to know one another.

At this time, your surgeon will also attempt to determine whether you are physically a good candidate for the procedure: would a face lift benefit you, and would any additional changes improve the overall result? He will also arrange for an evaluation of your general physical condition. He will undoubtedly describe for you in some detail what must be done before, during and after the operation, the results you can expect from it, and the possible complications.

When the surgeon has determined that you are a proper and reasonable candidate for a face lift and that his services can be of benefit to you, he will offer his care. If, at this point, you indicate that you want him to proceed, the bargain will be sealed.

At the first visit, the doctor may choose to show you preoperative and postoperative photographs of other patients. The plastic surgery community is divided on the wisdom of this procedure. Primarily, this is because the doctor, being human, is more likely to show you photographs of patients who have had what he considers good (rather than poor) results. Many physicians also feel that producing photos such as these implies a guarantee that the patient will have equally impressive results. However, no two people are the same. Skin types and bone structure vary enormously. Thin individuals with strong bones and thin skin have the most dramatic and remarkable results, while people with thicker skin and less prominent bone structure will have markedly less dramatic

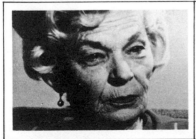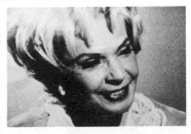

This prematurely aged woman underwent face lift and eyelid surgery. The results are self-evident. Not every patient changes so dramatically. Strong cheekbones add much to the result.

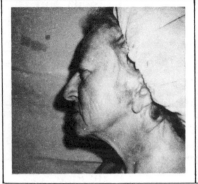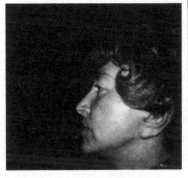

This woman underwent full face lift, eyelid surgery, and
rhinoplasty. The results are most pleasant. The nasal alteration
helps make up for absence of prominent cheekbones.

results in the hands of the same surgeon in the same set-
ting. It is therefore well to remember that the primary
purpose of photographs, if used, is merely to give you an
idea of what is done and how natural and improved the
patient appears some months after surgery. Photographs
also are useful in demonstrating the relative absence of
scarring in the face lift and certain other procedures.

At the first or second visit, the surgeon will take a series
of photographs of you, or arrange for a professional
photographer to do so. These photographs are important
in a number of ways. They are a graphic record of your
preoperative condition and are useful in postoperative
evaluation. They are also helpful in preoperative communication between surgeon and patient, in that they
make it easier to direct attention to various areas of difficulty. The photographs may also be valuable as a point
of reference. During surgery the patient is in a reclining
position, and the pull of gravity on excess skin is in a
different direction from what it is in the upright position.

The use of photographs, therefore, is often helpful in directing the surgeon's efforts.

After the first visit, the patient usually sees the doctor once again prior to surgery. This may be on a separate office visit during which photographs are reviewed and questions answered, or in the period immediately prior to surgery.

Whether the surgery is to be performed on an outpatient basis or in the hospital, you will be expected to follow several preoperative routines.

1. You will have a physical examination performed and a medical history taken by the hospital staff, the doctor's staff, or your personal physician. This is done in an effort to determine whether you have any infirmities which must be dealt with in order to maintain the high level of safety associated with the face lift procedure. The doctor also seeks to know whether you are taking any medications which might interfere with the medications to be used at surgery; whether you are allergic to any medications he might plan to use; whether you have had any significant illnesses which would alter or cancel his plans. He also needs to know certain basics such as your pulse rate and blood pressure in order to evaluate properly any changes that might occur before, during or after surgery. It is also important that he should know how well you heal after surgery and whether you have any tendency toward excessive bleeding. He will want to obtain other information which, when properly evaluated, can help protect you during surgery.

2. You will be advised to shampoo and shower with a prescribed antiseptic solution several times a day for 24 hours prior to surgery.

3. You will be advised to abstain from using aspirin or compounds containing aspirin for seventy-two hours prior to surgery, as these may promote bleeding.

4. You will be advised to abstain from alcohol for twenty-four hours prior to surgery.

5. You will be advised to take nothing by mouth later than midnight on the night prior to surgery and to have no breakfast or other food before the operation. The combination of drowsiness, from preoperative medication, and other factors may cause vomiting of food contents from the stomach. This may be inadvertently inhaled and lodged in the lungs, causing serious medical problems. Abstinence from food for eight hours prior to surgery reduces the likelihood of nausea and vomiting, and the chance of serious consequences if vomiting does take place.

THE FACE LIFT OPERATION

If your surgery is taking place in the hospital, you will be admitted one day prior to surgery. Your medical evaluation will take place at that time.

Approximately one hour prior to surgery, you will be given several medications by injection. These serve to relax you and often include a narcotic to combat pain. If your surgery is to be performed under local anesthesia, the preoperative sedation will be sufficiently strong to make you drowsy, if not downright sleepy. If your surgery is to be performed under general anesthesia, the preoperative medication will be considerably less powerful, since the general anesthesia will carry the load.

Prior to surgery, an intravenous (iv) tube will be installed in a vein in your arm. Through it you will be given fluids to maintain your level of hydration. This is necessary because you will not have eaten since midnight the previous night. The iv also serves as a conduit through which medications can be delivered without jabbing you constantly with hypodermics. The tube is removed shortly after surgery when you have recovered sufficiently to be able to take fluids by mouth.

In the operating room you will be placed, lying down, on the operating table, with your head and shoulders somewhat elevated. This is a comfortable position and is also a safety measure during surgery, since it helps to minimize bleeding. Your face and hair will be scrubbed with antiseptic solution. Face, neck and hair will then be painted and sprayed with another antiseptic solution, and you will be draped in a robe of sterile towels and sheets. Whether under general or local anesthesia, you will be aware of little or none of this. The area about the face and scalp will then be washed free of antiseptic solution, and indelible marks made in the area of the proposed incisions. The hair in this same area will be parted but not shaved. It has been demonstrated time and again that shaving of hair, which is unpleasant to the patient, is unnecessary from the standpoint of antiseptic technique.

If the operation is performed under local anesthesia, a solution of any one of a number of anesthetics will be used. Currently, the most common of these is lidocaine, a short-acting, relatively safe anesthetic about which a great deal is known. Several very fine pinpricks will be made in the facial skin for the introduction of local anesthetic. Because of the calming and pain-relieving effect of the medications already given, this part of the procedure is not particularly uncomfortable.

Face lift surgery takes approximately two hours. When

some other alteration is made in conjunction with it, additional time is required.

POSTOPERATIVE CARE

At the end of the procedure a large, well-padded, bulky dressing is placed over the face, head and neck. Care is taken to exclude the nose and mouth from the dressing. The eyes are most often left uncovered. Ice compresses are applied intermittently.

If you are an outpatient, the next four to six hours will be spent in a well monitored recovery area. In a hospital, they are spent in a room where supervision and monitoring are provided. At this point, the majority of the anesthetic will have worn off and you will be drowsy but able to function. There will be no pain. What little discomfort is experienced will usually be caused by the dressing and most patients are pleasantly surprised by the absence of postoperative pain.

When you leave the recovery facility for home or a convalescent facility, you will be advised that the large dressing will remain in place for twenty-four to forty-eight hours. After this, a lighter dressing may be applied. Sometimes no dressing is needed. You should remain in bed for the first twenty-four hours, except to use the bathroom. Thereafter, you may resume light activities.

In the first twenty-four hours, you will be advised to take no solid food, only fluids. Thereafter, there will be a gradual return to a soft diet. The purpose is to keep the patient from disturbing the postoperative result by moving the mouth vigorously in order to chew hard foods.

After forty-eight hours, you will be permitted to shower and shampoo with the same antiseptic solution used preoperatively. If you have been hospitalized, it is rarely necessary to remain in the hospital longer than forty-eight hours after surgery.

Between the second and fifth postoperative days, the sutures in front of the ears are removed. Your incision may be an irregular one running in front of your ear, with lines that dart in and out of the ear, or one that is entirely hidden within the ear. The choice depends on individual anatomy and on how your surgeon believes he can best disguise the resulting pencil-line scar.

By about the fourth or fifth postoperative day, your face will still be somewhat swollen. Areas of discoloration will persist, particularly around the neck. Between this time and the twelfth day, when the remaining sutures within the hairline are removed, the majority of swelling and discoloration will have disappeared.

Most patients are able to perform small chores and visit the supermarket toward the end of the first postoperative week. By the end of the second week, they are able to appear in public with more self-confidence. By the end of the third week, they should be able to disguise any remaining discoloration effectively enough to attend social functions.

In the immediate postsurgical period, medications are provided to deal with the occasional discomfort and sleeplessness associated with recovery. Antibiotics are usually not required.

POSTOPERATIVE DON'TS

1. Don't comb out your hair or use a hair dryer. This is because of the pulling effect of the comb on the sutures lines, and the possibility that the heat of the hair dryer might burn skin which has already been injured surgi-

cally. This is particularly to be guarded against because a certain degree of numbness persists in the area after surgery, and you therefore might injure yourself without feeling any warning pain. When you wash your hair during the first week, use an antiseptic shampoo.

2. Don't wear dangling or protruding earrings in pierced ear lobes. The ears, and particularly the ear lobes, remain numb for several months after a face lift, and it is easy to snag an earring and tear the ear lobe without being aware of it.

3. Don't apply hair color or processing until the physician declares you ready. This is usually between the third and fourth weeks.

4. Don't engage in vigorous physical activity during the first three postoperative weeks. This markedly increases blood pressure and may cause postoperative bleeding.

5. Don't bend over in such a fashion as to hang your head, since this can cause swelling or bleeding in the early postoperative period.

6. Don't sleep face down or lie flat in bed. Sleep on one or two pillows and on your back. This is to prevent postoperative swelling.

7. Don't use makeup near the incisions until your physician has advised you it is safe. This is usually about the tenth day.

8. Don't undergo facials or massage for three months after surgery.

9. Don't have sex for two weeks after surgery as physical activity and elevated blood pressure should be avoided in this period.

10. Don't expose yourself to direct sunlight. After three to four weeks, however, it is safe to appear in reflected sunlight. Even in these circumstances, it is important to

coat the operated area—in this case, the entire face—carefully with an effective sun block. Several of these agents are available without a prescription. The most effective ones contain paraaminobenzoic acid (PABA) or other identified active ingredients, such as benzophenones. To be effective, these agents must be applied several times daily. Additional care in the early postoperative period should include use of a large-brimmed hat and scrupulous avoidance of direct sunlight. After the first six weeks, exposure to the sun is less likely to damage the skin or cause significant swelling. This varies from individual to individual, however, and one must be prepared to avoid direct sunlight for periods of three to six months if that appears necessary.

PROBLEMS AND COMPLICATIONS

The overwhelming majority of problems known to be associated with face lift surgery are minor ones. The following discussion, however, includes all the minor and major problems known to occur in direct relationship to this surgery. As with all other forms of surgery, complications are usually less frequently experienced and less severe when surgery is performed by properly trained and experienced individuals.

The most common complication of face lift is hematoma (collection of blood under the skin). This has been estimated to occur in 7 percent of all patients undergoing face lift. However, this statistic should be interpreted in light of the fact that the overwhelming majority of these collections of blood are small, require no treatment, resolve by themselves in a matter of days, and in no way influence the ultimate result of the surgery. In a very small percentage of face lift patients with hematomas, however, the collection is of sufficient size to require secondary surgery. When hematomas occur after face lift surgery, they usually do so within the first twenty-four hours. Causes of this problem vary from hypertension to blood clotting disorders to inadequate control of bleeding during surgery.

Loss of small skin areas, primarily near suture lines, is also a reported complication. This is usually minor and self-limited.

Some surgeons report a temporary or permanent hair loss in the area of the scalp scar. This may be due to incision or suturing technique, to pulling the skin too tight, or perhaps to a hormonal reaction to surgery. In any event, it is usually a minor problem, is sometimes temporary and can be rectified.

The most serious complication associated with face lift surgery is injury to the facial nerve. This is the nerve that controls motion of the facial muscles. Bruising any branch of this nerve can produce weakness or loss of motion. Fortunately, this complication is extraordinarily rare. In most cases in which nerve injury does occur, it is temporary and self-limited. In a short time the patient returns to normal. If the nerve is actually cut, a repair at the time of surgery or at a later date can be performed.

Although accurate statistics on matters such as this are difficult to obtain, most surgeons do not encounter more than a few major complications in an entire lifetime of practice. You must know that these things occur, and you must enter into your surgery fully understanding not only what the procedure can do for you but the possibility, however minute, that problems could arise. In elective surgery such as the face lift, the fine, uncomplicated results so far overshadow the possibility of problems that it is unlikely that you will ever meet anyone who has experienced any of the complications we have just discussed.

LONG-TERM RESULTS

In the first postoperative days, it is difficult for the patient to evaluate the ultimate result of face lift surgery. Whether or not there is considerable swelling and discoloration, only the truly imaginative or experienced individual can at this time predict how successful the outcome will be. A "blue" period is common among patients at this point. This is often caused by the realization that the transformation is not instant or magical. This mood soon passes, and as the surgery matures the result is appreciated.

As the swelling recedes and the face regains its normal shape, a number of fine wrinkles which disappeared with early postoperative swelling may reappear. However, the face regains a more youthful, high-cheekboned, vital appearance. Over the first several postoperative months, there is an ever-so-slight daily change for the better. In evaluating this, it is important to realize that the objective of the operation has been to produce a graceful, more rested and youthful appearance, and not to pull the skin so tight that it shouts "face lift."

After two weeks, the incisions in front of the ear are somewhat pink, but are easily disguised with makeup. At three months, they are all but invisible.

At six months, the face lift will have matured, the memory of the surgery will have receded, and you will not be surprised when people tell you how well, how young or how rested you look.

You, yourself, will be the most critical judge of your surgery. When you see your surgeon for your six-month checkup, you will probably have forgotten your preoperative appearance. If you have become blasé and accustomed to your regained youthfulness, you will need only to compare your preoperative with postoperative photographs to appreciate once again the transformation.

Sometimes there are minor adjustments to be made in the postoperative period. This is not unusual, and you should be aware preoperatively of the possibility that such adjustments may be needed.

HOW LONG DOES A FACE LIFT LAST?

A face lift, like all other antiaging surgery, is directed at undoing the damage done by time. Nevertheless, the clock is always ticking. We all continue to age. This is not to say, however, that a face lift cannot have permanently beneficial effects.

Imagine the situation of twin sisters aged fifty. One decides to have her face lifted, the other does not. Immediately after surgery, sister No. 1 looks younger, more refreshed, and generally less burnt out than sister No. 2. As the years go on, however, both sisters continue to age. But even though sister No. 1 may notice, ten years after surgery, that she has a good deal of loose skin and an increasingly tired appearance, sister No. 2, who did not have a face lift, still looks considerably older than sister No. 1. In fact, sister No. 1, despite continuous aging, will always retain the edge in youthfulness created by her face lift.

One does not lose the benefit of a face lift. There is no sudden falling of the face. But, we cannot stop the clock.

CHAPTER 3

THREE OTHER WAYS
TO IMPROVE YOUR FACE

Although the face lift and eyelid operations are the most important procedures employed to correct the damage caused by aging, a number of other approaches are now being used. Among these are chemical peeling, dermabrasion, and cheekbone implants.

CHEMICAL FACE PEELING

Face peeling, or chemosurgery, is a process through which the skin is rejuvenated by the application of a combination of chemicals. These chemicals produce a burn-like reaction, and result in the removal of the superficial layers of the skin. This method, whether applied by cosmeticians, dermatologists or plastic surgeons, has been used for many years in the treatment of fine facial wrinkles, abnormal pigmentation, and superficial acne scars. Skin peeling is potentially dangerous and should be done by properly trained personnel only.

Chemical face peeling may be used alone or in combination with facial surgery. The usual reasons for the addition of chemical face peeling to such surgery are fine wrinkles around the mouth and cheeks, crow's-feet alongside the eyelids and fine lines in the forehead.

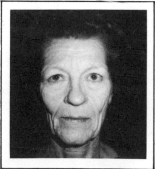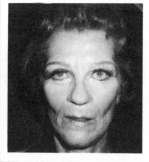

This woman had extensive fine wrinkling of the facial skin.
She underwent blepharoplasty and chemical face peel.

Despite its various uses, chemical peeling is best reserved for the treatment of fine wrinkles, where its effects are most predictable. Although many physicians have reported fine results using chemical peel to treat other abnormalities of the skin, many of these, particularly those involving treatment of pigment changes of the facial skin after pregnancy, are unfortunately not easy to duplicate. Therefore, except in special circumstances, chemical peeling is reserved for the treatment of facial aging not responsive to surgical techniques, or for use instead of surgery.

Phenol is the active ingredient of the majority of chemical peeling solutions. In the United States, the most frequently used combination is a mixture of phenol, croton oil and other ingredients.

The patient about to undergo chemical face peeling is prepared much as she would be for cosmetic surgery. The procedure is carried out in the doctor's office suite or hospital. The patient is advised to refrain from eating breakfast prior to the chemosurgery. Sedation and pain killers are given preoperatively.

After the patient has been sedated or anesthetized, as the case may be, the skin is prepared with a surgical soap. It is then cleansed thoroughly with an ether solution. This serves to eliminate the oil that normally accumulates in the lubricating glands of the skin, and allows a more effective application of the chemical agents during the procedure.

The solution is applied uniformly, using ordinary cotton applicators. The skin is stroked lightly with the solution until a frosty white appearance develops. At this point, the patient may experience a mild burning sensation.

This disappears in minutes. This limited discomfort is due to the anesthetic quality of phenol.

Care is taken to keep the solution from dripping. The line of application is gradually feathered as the area of treatment is exceeded. This is particularly important in areas of the face where there is no natural line of definition. This technique is used in treatment of lines around the mouth, since these lead eventually to the lower portion of the jaw and the area beneath the chin. The solution is gradually applied in decreasing and feathered amounts to the area of skin beneath the chin. This makes for a gradual change in skin texture. Where there is a natural skin crease such as the nasolabial line, the application of the chemical agent stops there.

The most common area for application of chemical peel is around the mouth. Vertical lines in the upper lip and circular and horizontal lines of the chin and lower lip are not responsive to other therapeutic means. These lines can be a significant problem, even when a full face lift is being performed. In such cases, chemical peeling or dermabrasion (another approach to smoother skin that will also be described in this chapter) is an important adjunct.

The most difficult place to deal with is the border of the lips, where the deep lines cross the pigmented area. This region is particularly troublesome because lipstick and other cosmetics may run through the furrows and produce an objectionable appearance. Great care is taken in attempting to deal with these areas adequately. The chemical peel serves to improve, but not entirely remove the problem.

After the solution has been applied to the face, a mask

of waterproof adhesive tape is applied directly to the skin. Care is taken to leave the eyebrows, eyes, nostrils and mouth exposed. The tape is applied in small units in order to cover the area in question accurately. Approximately six to eight hours after the application of the tape mask, the face becomes quite swollen. The eyelids frequently swell shut. This is what is normally expected. The mask is left in position for approximately forty-eight hours. The patient is instructed not to talk unnecessarily, and to keep the face as immobile as possible, in order not to disturb the mask and the underlying burn. Liquids are taken through a straw, pain medications are provided, and the patient is advised to keep the head elevated and to remain in bed resting.

After twenty-four hours, some fluid may weep from beneath the mask. The swelling is constant, and somewhat frightening in appearance, at this stage. After forty-eight hours, the patient returns to the doctor's office, where the adhesive tape mask is removed. This may be painful, and some patients require the use of an analgesic beforehand.

After the tape mask is removed, the skin is red, moist and clearly injured. The surface resembles that of a second-degree burn. The treated surfaces are gently dusted with thymol iodide powder, a soothing bacteriostatic agent which is applied either with a cotton-tipped applicator or a salt shaker. Within twenty-four hours after the removal of the mask, the thymol iodide adheres to the surface, and a golden-brown crust is formed. The powder is applied generously three times daily over the next three days.

Five to seven days following the peel, an ointment is

applied over the crust to soften it and hasten its separation from the face. Usually, plain Vaseline®, A&D®, or antibiotic ointment is used.

Approximately seven days after the peel, the entire crust falls away, and ordinary gentle washing of the face with soap and water is encouraged. However, there must be no attempt to actively remove what crust remains. At this point, many physicians use a steroid cream to reduce inflammation and soften the treated area.

From the seventh to the twenty-first days following the peel, the skin takes on a red and somewhat granular appearance. This is normal, and nothing can be done to prevent it.

Most patients can wear cosmetics by the fourteenth day. By the end of the first month, the pinkness about the face begins to recede noticeably. The skin texture returns to normal, and at the end of three months both color and quality of the skin should be close to normal.

It is important to maintain certain precautions for up to six months following skin peel. Since the chemical peelant removes a great deal of the melanin in the basal layers of the skin, a large proportion of the skin's protection against the sun's rays has been lost. Therefore, patients are advised to avoid both direct and reflected sunlight for up to six months. This is especially important during the middle of the day and is even more so in tropical and subtropical climates The patient must wear a wide-brimmed hat and a suitable sun block or sun-screening agent. The most effective sun-blocking agents contain paraaminobenzoic acid, oxybenzone or dioxybenzone. They are available without a prescription, easy to apply and pleasant in texture and fragrance.

Chemical face peel is useful when applied in the proper circumstances. It is not without complications, however. Those most commonly encountered include milia, or whitehead pimples; increased sensitivity of the skin to sunlight; reduction in skin pigmentation, usually in an irregular fashion; deep burns or scar formation; and prolonged redness of the skin. Fortunately, the complication rate has been low when the procedure has been performed upon properly selected patients.

Chemical face peeling is most effective in individuals with fair skin and minimal pigmentation. It is least effective and most dangerous when applied to individuals with oily, dark skin who have spent many years constantly exposed to the elements. Therefore, the patient best served by chemical face peeling is the fair-skinned individual with fine facial wrinkles. Whether this is the method of choice is a decision to be made by the patient and her surgeon.

DERMABRASION

Dermabrasion is the mechanical removal of superficial layers of the skin down to the deep layer or dermis. Usually a rotating wire brush or abrasive cylinder, driven by an electric motor, is used. Dermabrasion is used to alter scars, remove tattoos and fine wrinkles, and assist in the surgical smoothing of acne-scarred skin. The procedure is performed under local or general anesthesia. The skin is made taut either by injection or by manual pressure. The rotating brush or drum is applied to the skin until the proper depth is achieved. Great care must be taken to avoid damaging the deep structures of the dermis. This would result in healing by scar formation, rather than the production of fine new skin.

Postoperatively, the site of dermabrasion is uncomfortable. It is covered with blood and crust for several days. This gradually peels away and pink new skin appears. Various ointments and creams are applied to help soften and protect the new skin.

Dermabrasion is an effective agent when properly applied. However, it is difficult to achieve good results from this technique in areas which are not essentially flat and firm. Therefore, dermabrasion is most often confined to the cheeks, forehead and large body surfaces.

The most frequent use of dermabrasion is on acne-scarred skin. Here the rotating brush or cylinder acts to flatten the edges of the skin pits, making them less unsightly and the skin smoother. This is often done in conjunction with some variant of the face lift operation, which helps to tighten and smooth the cheek skin. This combination also reduces shadows formed by the pits and scars, thus enhancing the result.

Another common use of dermabrasion is in the removal of tattoos. Dermabrasion removes the upper layer, or epidermis, and exposes tattoo pigment lying within the dermis. The application of wet dressings helps to draw out the colors. The procedure is repeated several times and can result in the thorough destruction of the tattoo. Although, unfortunately, there is often a noticeable difference in skin texture, and visible scarring results, many patients find this more acceptable than the tattoo.

CHEMICAL PEEL OR DERMABRASION?

Dermabrasion and chemical face peeling have many points of similarity: the method of healing, the need for precautions against exposure to the sun, and some possible complications, including development of milia, redness of the skin and scarring. Laboratory studies have shown, however, that the histological (cellular) changes induced by the two methods may be different. The main finding of importance to the patient is the fact that following chemical peel there appears to be an increase in the amount of elastic tissue in the deeper levels of the skin. This is not the case after dermabrasion, and could conceivably explain why there is a greater benefit in the treatment of fine wrinkles following chemical face peel, than there is with dermabrasion. On the other hand, the use of chemical face peeling for the treatment of acne scarring has been disappointing. We have, through experience, come to realize that both of these useful procedures must be carefully applied to selected patients and selected problems in order to be properly beneficial.

CHEEKBONE AND CHIN IMPLANTS

Cheekbones are an important element in facial beauty. Flat, non-rounded cheeks are less attractive than high, prominent, rounded ones. Because of this, many patients request that the plastic surgeon give them a high-cheekboned look.

The face lift, as we have seen, very commonly produces a return to an appearance in which the cheekbones appear more prominent. However, in patients who did not when young have this attractive characteristic, and also in patients who wish to heighten it even more than is possible with a face lift, another approach can be used. This is known as cheekbone augmentation.

Surgeon and patient determine preoperatively the area and extent of the correction to be made with the aid of small, commercially produced cheekbone implants. These are made, in various shapes and sizes, of hard silicone rubber. They are inserted, under local or general anesthesia, and are secured in place by sutures. Insertion is done either through an incision beneath the lower lashes or from the inside of the mouth. The access route depends on a number of factors, including the preference of the surgeon.

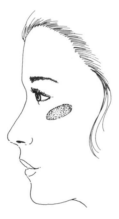

The general position and appearance
of cheek bone implants.

Some discomfort is felt during the first twenty-four to forty-eight hours following this procedure, but actual pain is minimal. Antibiotics are usually used. Considerable swelling is found in the area of surgery for several weeks. This gradually resolves, revealing the sought-after result. Chin augmentation also produces dramatic results. It is very simply performed and is discussed in the chapter on nasal surgery.

Difficulties most commonly associated with this operation are poor positioning or slippage of the implant, and infection. In either case, the implant must be removed, but can be replaced at a later date.

CHAPTER 4

A YOUTHFUL LOOK
AROUND YOUR EYES

Your eyes are the most important feature of your face. The condition of the skin around them therefore has a particularly significant effect on the way other people see you. Unfortunately, the eyelids usually acquire an "older" appearance before other facial features show the effects of aging. Many patients also have other eye-area problems such as deep frown lines between the eyebrows, or excessively overhanging eyebrows. It is gratifying to report that help is available for individuals who want to have such conditions corrected, and that many people today are benefiting from plastic surgery directed to this part of the face.

WHAT CAUSES EYELID WRINKLES AND BAGS?

The skin on the eyelids, upper and lower, is the thinnest skin on your face. It is also very loose. It is not firmly bound to the underlying bones and muscles. Delicate and fragile in appearance, it is a mirror of your relationship to your environment and emotions, and also of your time of life.

The skin of the eyelid is the first to be affected by allergy, irritation, unhappiness, sunburn, overindulgence or lack of sleep. It responds by repeated stretching, wrinkling and shrinking. Finally, with aging, it is no longer able to shrink back to size. This is because it has lost some of the elastic fibers which, in youth, allowed it to bounce back after stretching.

When eyelid skin is stretched by various activities and aged both naturally and by sunlight, cigarettes and alcohol, it very early loses its youthful elasticity. This sets the stage for baggy, wrinkled lower eyelids and excessively heavy, hanging, sleepy-looking upper eyelids. In most individuals, the muscle beneath the eyelid skin begins to thin out and stretch. As a result, packets of fatty tissue which normally surround the eyeball begin to poke out through the weakened muscle and produce baggy, puffy eyelids.

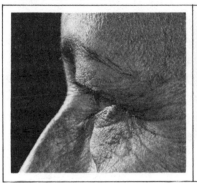 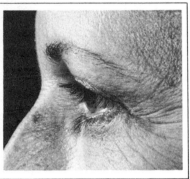

| Before: Notice the prominent *bags* beneath the lower eyelids. | After: The result six months after upper and lower lid blepharoplasty. Note absence of *bags*. |

Aging and stretching of tissue are the most common ways to acquire baggy eyelids. Less frequently, plastic surgeons see young people, even teen-agers, with the most profound and unsightly pouches beneath their eyes. In these cases, it is usually a family trait. As a rule, however, bagginess of the lower eyelids, heaviness of the upper eyelids, excessively wrinkled skin on the upper and lower eyelids, and deepening crow's-feet and laugh lines are the first signs of aging about the face. In fact, the eyelids usually age long before other facial features. It is for this reason that eyelid surgery is frequently performed on patients who, although not yet candidates for face lift, are beginning to look tired beyond their years. Because of this, and because the surgical solution to this problem has been overwhelmingly successful, eyelid surgery is probably the procedure most often performed by plastic surgeons today.

HOW EYELID SURGERY IS DONE

The technical name for eyelid surgery, *blepharoplasty*, is derived from the Greek. Roughly translated, it means "to mold the eyelids," which is precisely what it does. Blepharoplasty has few complications and is relatively painless. Recovery is rapid, and results are very long lasting. The operation can be performed in outpatient surgical facilities or private operating suites, or in hospital operating rooms. Each year, more and more blepharoplasties are carried out on an outpatient basis. General anesthesia is rarely used. In most parts of the United States, the operation is performed using preoperative sedation, a sort of twilight sleep usually produced by use of intravenous Valium® or other tranquilizer, and analgesics, prior to surgery. Local anesthetics are then used in small quantities around the eyelids. The operation takes about one hour to perform.

Prior to surgery, with the patient in a sitting position, the upper eyelids are carefully marked in such a way as to indicate the amount of skin that must be removed. After the patient is anesthetized, the excess skin of the upper eyelid, and the protruding fat which has made the upper eyelids heavy, are removed. Bleeding is controlled by the use of electrocautery. The skin is closed with tiny silk or nylon sutures. A similar procedure is carried out on the lower eyelids.

The incision in the lower eyelid is made just beneath the lower eyelashes. (Care is taken not to disturb the eyelashes themselves.) This results in a very fine and ultimately invisible line. The incision in the upper eyelid is placed to fall in the skin crease with the eyes open, and becomes all but invisible when the eyes are shut.

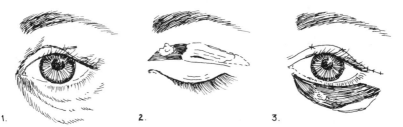

1.   2.   3.

Figure 1: Aging upper and lower eyelids. Figure 2: The removal of excess skin and protruding pockets of fat from the upper eyelids. Figure 3: The upper incision closed and the excess skin and fat being removed from the lower lid.

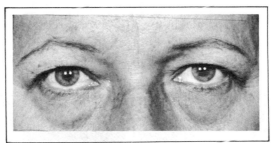

Forty-seven year old woman with marked overhang of the upper eyelids and *bags* of the lower eyelids.

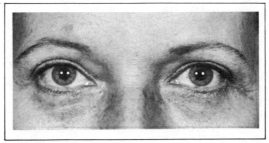

Six months after blepharoplasty. Note the wider appearance of eyes. Upper lids and eyelashes visible. *Bags* removed.

Great care must be taken during the surgery to remove enough skin and fat for an effective and graceful cosmetic improvement, but at all costs the surgeon must avoid removing too much skin, which can result in an unattractive and unnatural look. Here, there is no substitute for a well-trained and experienced plastic surgeon. If you are having a blepharoplasty, your timetable might consist of early morning surgery followed by several hours of resting in bed on your back, with constant application of ice-soaked gauze pads or Gel-ice packs. This serves to control swelling in the immediate postsurgical period. After several hours, you are permitted to walk to the bathroom and take liquids. Painkillers are given by mouth or by injection to control any minor discomfort. The use of ice compresses is continued for approximately twenty-four hours.

The patient returns home or to the hospital room or con-

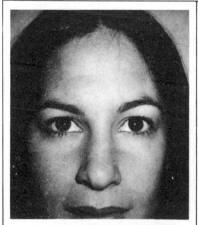

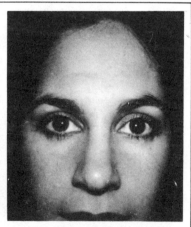

A twenty-five year
old woman with congenitally
heavy upper eyelids.

Five months after surgery the
upper eyelids are finer
and the eyes appear more alert.

valescent facility, and remains quietly in bed for as much of the first twenty-four hours as possible. In the second twenty-four hours, ice may be discontinued and activities and diet may be increased. At this point, little or no pain or discomfort is felt.

Although routines vary among surgeons, most patients are permitted to resume all activities, including use of eye makeup, by the seventh to tenth postoperative day. By this time swelling and discoloration have disappeared.

COMPLICATIONS

Very few complications are known to be associated with blepharoplasty. The most common complaint from patients is that not enough skin was removed. Sometimes this is true, but most often the surgeon has exercised good judgment in not overdoing skin removal and putting the patient at risk.

A serious and fairly frequently seen complication is called ectropion. This is a condition, usually in the lower eyelid, in which either too much skin has been removed or the patient has had some unforeseen postoperative swelling or bleeding. As a result, the eyelid is lifted away from the eye. This is usually temporary, and can easily be reversed by simple measures. When the problem is severe, there are numerous minor surgical techniques for correcting it. Ectropion is a complication you should know about, but is rare indeed in the hands of properly prepared individuals.

The most common complications of eyelid surgery are either excessive tearing or temporary lack of tears in the early post-operative period. This is an annoyance which can be dealt with by local means. It usually resolves spontaneously. Another difficulty, is development of small pimples or milia in stitch areas. These require un-roofing with a sterile needle and moist packs.

In blepharoplasty, as in all other surgical procedures, there have been reports over the years of various disasters, including several cases of blindness. It is fair to say, however, that one assumes a greater risk, statistically, of significant complications when undergoing a tonsilectomy than a blepharoplasty. Eyelid surgery is a well-tolerated operation in which the results are immediately visible and appreciated, and carries minimal risk.

ONE OR TWO PROCEDURES?

By the time most people have experienced sufficient facial aging to make them consider a face lift, the eyelids are usually more than ready to benefit from blepharoplasty. Although eyelid surgery is often done separately, it is just as commonly performed as part of a total overhaul of the face. In the shop talk of plastic surgery, the phrase *face and eyes* is used to refer to an approach in which a face lift and blepharoplasty are accomplished in a single trip to the operating room.

The patient will obtain greatest benefit if the various parts of the face are in harmony. It seems foolish to have face lift surgery to produce a smooth, youthful face while neglecting tired-looking eyelids. Usually, we counsel a patient planning a face lift to consider having eyelid surgery at the same time.

THE BROW LIFT

If a patient has excessively overhanging eyebrows, a "brow lift" is sometimes performed. In this operation, a wedge of skin above the eyebrows is removed, and the eyebrows are then placed in a more taut and higher posi-

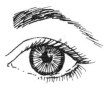

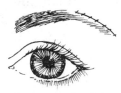

(A) A slightly drooped eyebrow.

(B) The brow after lifting by removal of a wedge of skin above the brow.

tion, giving the eyes a more open and less haggard look. The incision is barely perceptible. Most of our patients who have undergone this surgery say they believe the scar is not significant enough to detract from the dramatic change in their appearance.

FROWN LINES

Many patients complain to the plastic surgeon of deep, vertical frown lines over the bridge of the nose, between the eyebrows. Such furrows are caused by excessive use

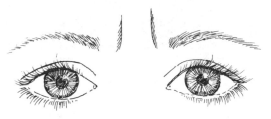

(A) Vertical *frown* lines between the eyebrows.

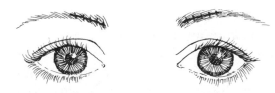

(B) The placement of incisions within the brow, and the result. In reality, results are impressive but not as perfect as in the stylized drawing.

of several small muscles, including the corrugator muscle of the brow.

To correct frown lines, a small incision is made within the eyebrow and a section of muscle is removed. No hair is shaved. The procedure produces little or no noticeable scarring, and depth of the furrows is greatly reduced. The operation also impedes the ability to frown and, hence, to form the unsightly lines once again.

In the past, lines were sometimes filled in with minute amounts of medical-grade liquid silicone. Use of this substance is currently forbidden by law.

EAST AND WEST

An exceedingly popular eyelid operation in Asia, and in some areas of the United States, is a procedure in which Oriental eyes are converted to Western eyes.

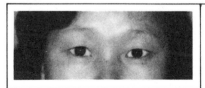
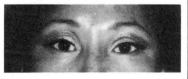

The surgical change from *Oriental* upper eyelids,
to *Western* upper eyelids.

An Oriental upper eyelid does not have the mid-eyelid fold which is characteristic of the Western eyelid. This is because a small wisp of muscle which attaches to the skin of the Western eyelid is absent in the Oriental lid. By simply making an incision in the upper lid and joining this muscle to the skin, a fold is created and the eyes appear more fully open, in the Western fashion.

Some patients, on the other hand, wish to have their eyes assume a more almond-shaped or cat-like appearance. Surgeons may produce this by excising skin in the outside areas of each eyelid and performing a temporal lift.

WHEN IS IT TIME TO CORRECT SIGNS OF AGING?

The time to consider cosmetic surgery of the face and eyelids is when changes caused by aging have become a visible and unpleasant part of your appearance. Just when this occurs, of course, will vary from person to person; but the usual age range at which one may become aware of the problem is forty-five to fifty-five years. When these changes make surgery a consideration, there is no advantage in waiting until sagging is more pronounced. That produces years of looking old while feeling young, and is entirely unjustified.

Having a face lift at the age at which you first think it necessary does not mean that you will require additional surgery, or more surgery than if you had waited until your condition became intolerable. Often individuals who have a face lift performed in their middle to late forties need little more than a slight touch up many years later. It should also be noted that there is no reasonable limit to the number of times the procedure can be performed, nor the age at which it may be performed. As skin loosens, stretches and becomes unsightly, it can be removed, and this procedure can be repeated whenever necessary.

To check on whether you may be ready for a face lift, stand before a mirror, place your open palms against your cheekbones and temples, and lift upward. If your face rises and looks instantly more youthful and pleasant, you may be one of those who could benefit from a face lift. Of course, the change produced by lifting with the hands is not precisely the same as that produced by a surgical face lift. However, lifting with the hands will give you some idea of the type of effect that can be obtained surgically. While still in front of your mirror, you should also check for excess folds of skin hanging over your upper eyelids; drooping of the outside of the eyebrows; bags and wrinkles beneath the eyes; deep nasolabial folds; fine vertical lines and wrinkles around the mouth; jowls; and loose neck skin or vertical bands in the neck. When this is done, you will have gone through a plastic surgeon's checklist. Usually a combination of several of these signs indicates aging of the face, of the type that would benefit from a face lift and/or eyelid surgery.

The following chart is intended for self-evaluation and general information. All of the signs of facial aging listed there have been discussed in preceding chapters.

Beside the name of each problem is the name of the procedure best suited to correct it. As you check the areas of particular concern to you and refer to the corrective measures opposite, you will find that the same measure often applies to several problems. This reinforces the general belief among plastic surgeons that isolated temporal lifts or neck lifts are rarely indicated, and that most often the patient's interests are best served by a full face lift, plus whatever ancillary measures might be benficial.

TWENTY SIGNS OF FACIAL AGING AND HOW THEY CAN BE CORRECTED

Problems	Appropriate Corrective Procedures
1. Heavy upper eyelids	Blepharoplasty. Results usually excellent.
2. Excess, overhanging upper eyelid skin	Blepharoplasty. Results usually excellent.

3. Baggy lower eyelids	Blepharoplasty. Results usually excellent.
4. Dark rings under eyes	Cannot be completely corrected, but blepharoplasty smooths skin and reduces the shadows caused by baggy lower eyelids, thereby reducing the dark appearance without actually removing the pigmented skin.
5. Drooping eyebrows	A temporal lift may be adequate in mild cases. A brow lift removes a small amount of skin directly above the eyebrow and effectively lifts the eyebrow, leaving a relatively unnoticeable scar.
6. Deep horizontal lines on the forehead	Surgical procedures to correct this depend on destroying motion in a portion of the frontalis muscle of the forehead. These procedures effectively eliminate or reduce deep horizontal lines, but also reduce or eliminate expression in the forehead as well as ability to lift one's eyebrows. They are recommended, therefore, under special circumstances. Other treatments include electric coagulation of the lines, or injection of small amounts of medical-grade liquid silicone (not legally available at this time) in order to reduce the depth of these lines.
7. Vertical frown lines between the eyes	Small incisions within the eyebrow allow the surgeon to cut the corrugator muscle, reducing the ability to produce this frown. Liquid silicone in small amounts (not legally available at this

	time) also helps to reduce these lines.
8. Horizontal frown line between the eyes	A small incision in the frown line permits cutting of the procerus muscle, which helps reduce production of this frown. Small amounts of liquid silicone (not legally available at this time) also help reduce the depth of this line.
9. Crow's-feet	Cannot be eliminated. These are normal side-effects of having an animated face. They can be lessened somewhat by a temporal lift, face lift or chemical peel.
10. Deep nasolabial crease from nose to corners of mouth	Can be improved, but not eliminated, by face lift.
11. Loss of cheek substance	Usually fat pads in the cheeks which have drifted downward on the face can be replaced in more youthful position by a face lift. This can also be accomplished by insertion of silicone rubber cheek implants either through eyelid incisions or through the mouth. Results can be quite dramatic.
12. Jowls	A face lift can give excellent results.
13. Deep line from corner of mouth to jowls	These lines run in the same general direction as, but below, the nasolabial creases. They can be improved, but not completely eliminated, by a face lift.
14. Fine vertical lines around mouth and lips	These lines are not affected by a face lift. They can be significantly improved by a chemical peel.

15. Enlarged, hanging earlobes	These are a common sign of aging. They can be corrected by simple excision of a portion of the lobe, alone or with a face lift.
16. Vertical bands in front of the neck	A face lift and a secondary incision beneath the chin will usually correct this problem, which is most often caused by loose bands of platysma muscle.
17. Deep horizontal lines around the neck	A face lift is usually effective. Sometimes a low horizontal incision is used, in addition, to remove some excess neck skin and improve the result.
18. Turkey gobbler neck	A face lift and an additional Z-shaped incision under the chin usually correct this problem.
19. Double chin	An incision under the chin and removal of fat, often with chin enlargement, yields good results.
20. "No" chin	Such a problem is usually accentuated by aging. It is easily corrected by a face lift and chin enlargement.

THE MINI LIFT

Perhaps this is a good place to deal with something known rather mysteriously as the "mini lift." To most plastic surgeons, the mini lift is a source of annoyance. It has been in and out of fashion over the years, but whatever its social status, it has never been a good operation. We have found that when patients request a mini lift they are never quite sure of what the term means, and in fact are not adequately informed, concerning the plastic surgery which they are seeking. The inventor of what is known as the mini lift may well have been a pioneer

French cosmetic surgeon, Madame Noël, who practiced in Paris in the early part of the twentieth century. Madame Noël, among others, is credited with removing a small amount of skin in front of the ears and pulling the cheeks tight with sutures. By today's standards, this is inexcusably minimal surgery. The yield is nothing more than a temporary tightening of the cheek skin. The results are neither significant nor permanent. Today's face lift surgery, whether a full face lift or a temporal lift, includes the lifting of the skin with its padding off the underlying structures so that it can be cleanly redraped and bound by healing into its new position.

Most plastic surgeons believe that a mini lift gives mini results. A simple tuck is not adequate to correct true aging of the facial tissues. Beware of miracle cures. There are many disreputable purveyors of plastic surgical "snake oil" today, and the intelligent consumer should be on guard against them.

You will notice from your evaluation of the chart presented in this chapter that unless your complaint is merely a wrinkle of skin in front of your ear, what is commonly known as a mini lift will not suffice. Unfortunately, however, some confusion stems from the fact that many well-meaning advisors, as well as some plastic surgeons, refer to the temporal lift as a mini lift. We hope that our discussion has made clear the differences between the two.

CHAPTER 5

IMPROVING YOUR NOSE

You may call it a nose job or nose bob. Plastic surgeons call it a nasoplasty or rhinoplasty. The word *rhinoplasty* comes from the Greek, and means a molding of the nose. Whatever term is used, this is the procedure that brought plastic surgery into the twentieth century, an operation that has been performed often enough in the last quarter of a century to make it a household word.

Cosmetic surgery of the nose was begun in the early part of this century by a German surgeon, Jacques Joseph. Dr. Joseph developed a method of removing a portion of the bone in a large and unattractive-looking nose. He soon published his results and gathered about him a group of adventurous and interested young surgeons from all over the world, who learned and expanded on the Joseph techniques and brought them back to their native countries. This technique was rapidly accepted, and gradually improved upon, in America.

At one time, many "nose jobs" were rather obvious looking. Over the years, however, increased experience and free exchange of ideas have enabled plastic surgeons to learn to produce much more graceful and natural-looking noses. The first nasoplasty operation was developed to reduce the size of the nose. Now, techniques have evolved to the point at which we can not only make noses smaller but can selectively thin them, refine them, turn them up, push them back and, in some cases, even make them larger.

Plastic surgery, however, is more than just technique. Basic to everything we can achieve is a sense of art, balance, and grace. Very often, in evaluating a patient's facial features, we find that the nose is not the offending feature. The face, and particularly the face in profile, is a balance of features. To look at the nose alone is to miss the forest for the trees. A strong and projecting chin can balance a large nose. A weak and receding chin can make even an average-sized nose appear outlandishly prominent. Unfortunately, individuals with large noses very commonly have weak or small chins. This magnifies the problem.

In the early years of nasal surgery, when a rhinoplasty would be performed the patient would be improved, but something would be missing from the result. Today, we know what the problem was. We know that a large percentage of patients undergoing nasal surgery can also benefit greatly from having their chins enlarged.

To see the importance of a balance between nose and chin, flip through the pages of any fashion magazine. Look at any of the models you consider beautiful. Their

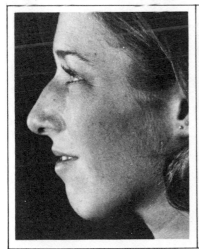

A twenty-five year old woman prior to rhinoplasty.

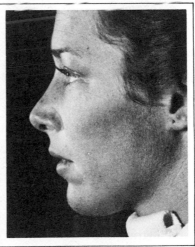

Six months after rhinoplasty and chin augmentation, the result is a balanced, graceful and more attractive profile.

features, individually, may not be perfect, and many do not have perfect noses, but all have strong, prominent chins, which balance the noses. While you are looking, make a note of the fact that all these "beautiful people" have prominent cheekbones as well. In fact, strong cheekbones and a strong chin may give the illusion of beauty in spite of other features that are less than perfect. It is important, therefore, if you are considering a rhinoplasty, to look at your nose as an integral part of your face, not as an isolated feature.

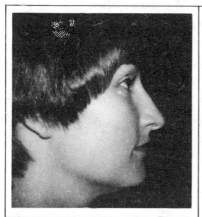

Before rhinoplasty.

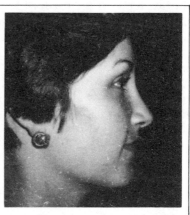

Notice the graceful facial balance after rhinoplasty.

PROFILE ANALYSIS

A well-known artistic rule of thumb, based on the work of the nineteenth century sculptor, Schadow, is used in evaluating the geometry of the face. In this method, the face, from the eyebrows to the bottom of the chin, is divided into six sections. The first three equal parts begin at the eyebrow and end at the bottom of the nose. The next includes the upper lip; the last two, the lower lip and the jaw. The perfect contour is represented by a line

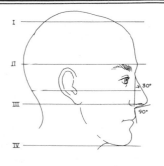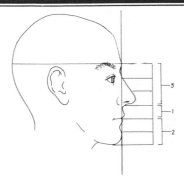

(A) From Schadow, the accepted angle between nose and lip, 90–95°; between nose and face, 30°.

(B) Face divided into sections and illustrates line from forehead to chin in *perfect* profile.

from the forehead at the level of the eyebrows which drops as a perpendicular and is touched by the chin. Add to this analysis an angle between the upper lip and the nose of 90 to 95 degrees, and a straight nasal dorsum or bridge, and the result is a perfect, if uninteresting, profile. Individuals, fortunately, do not conform exactly to this mold. Nevertheless, this is the basic facial balance that represents beauty in our society. Through understand-

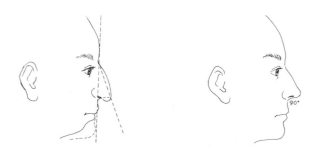

Profile correction according to the profile analysis in previous illustration. A similar but less severe analysis is made by the plastic surgeon in planning nasal surgery.

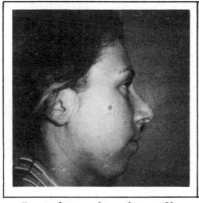
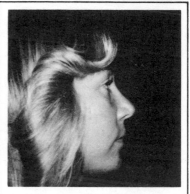

| By understanding the profile analysis, nasal and chin surgery may be planned. | Six months after surgery a more balanced and attractive profile results. |

ing, on this ideal level, what makes a profile or a face appealing, a clearer idea of what to strive for has been developed. However, it is also valuable to realize that harmony of the facial features is important, and that a natural and graceful overall appearance is far more desirable than a perfect feature.

HAVING YOUR NOSE DONE

If you should decide that you might benefit from some alteration in the appearance of your nose, you will no doubt make an appointment with a plastic surgeon. In his office, he will seek to understand your motivation for this change, and try to assure himself that you are a realistic as well as a well-motivated patient. He will analyze your nose and your facial features and will answer questions related to your individual circumstances. At this visit, the surgeon may choose to show you a series of preoperative and postoperative photos of other patients. If this is done, it is in no way intended as a suggestion that you, your nose or anything about you will look like the patient in question. The intention is to show representative examples of what can be done, and not to imply any sort of guarantee.

Most surgeons will attempt to demonstrate to you what changes are advisable in your case, either with sketches or by altering photographs of your profile so as to represent the changes planned at surgery. There must be give-and-take during this procedure. You must actively participate and make your feelings known. This is the time to communicate your wishes to your surgeon and to arrive at an understanding of what is to be done. In most cases, the surgeon can deliver a good approximation of what he sets out to do. However, he cannot help you to look the way you wish to look if you do not help him to understand your desires.

This session is also a time at which the surgeon can tell you what is, or is not, possible. The same changes are not always feasible in every case. For example, there is no way in which a large, bulbous, thick-skinned nose can be transformed into a fine, thin and perfect feature. There is a need, therefore, for good communication on the part of the surgeon, and a realistic understanding of the procedure on the part of the patient.

WHAT ABOUT THE CHIN?

During this period of initial analysis, many people are shocked to find the surgeon suggesting improvement of the jawline. Once the principles of profile analysis are explained, most patients understand more fully but are still not wholly receptive to the idea. Many are thinking, "What? Something else is wrong with me?" and then resist. Hopefully communication will be good enough to convince the patient to consider this additional change.

If you should decide to ask the surgeon to add projection to your chin, you will be glad to know that this is a relatively minor procedure. It is usually carried out with rhinoplasty, but may be done as a separate operation, and is usually done on an outpatient basis.

The operation requires local anesthesia and the insertion

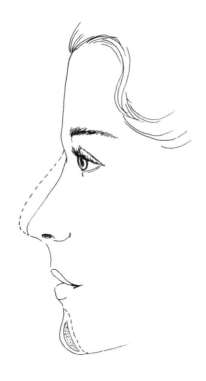

A nasal reduction and chin
enlargement. The chin
implant is represented by
a stippled area.

of a small, shaped, silicone unit which fits smoothly against your jaw. The implant is inserted through a small incision at the very bottom of the inside of the lower lip, or through a small incision under the chin. In either case, scarring is minimal and the major complaint is one of discomfort during the first few days after surgery. Heavy elastic bandages are used to reduce swelling and keep the implant in its proper position. These are removed during the first week, at which time a marked improvement, though not the final result, can be seen.

The first several weeks after chin augmentation are accompanied by swelling in the area. The normal depression between the lower lip and the chin is temporarily lost, and the lower portion of the face is larger than usual. This may not be noticeable to others, but it will be a source of annoyance to you. Gradually, your tolerance builds and the swelling recedes, and soon the only thing noticeable is the graceful projection of the new chin. The stitches are removed from the skin during the first week, and in several months the scar beneath the chin fades and disappears. If the incision is inside the mouth, there will be no noticeable scar.

The complications associated with this procedure are minimal. When they occur, the most common complaints are improper positioning of the implant, and rarely an infection around the implant. In the case of improper positioning, the chin implant is removed and repositioned. In the case of infection, the implant is removed and then reinserted after a six-week waiting period. In general, chin augmentation is a very low-risk procedure. The results are almost uniformly good, and are usually greatly appreciated because the patient was not fully aware of what a remarkable improvement could be produced by this small procedure.

THE RHINOPLASTY

A rhinoplasty may be performed either in the hospital or in an outpatient operating suite. It is almost universally performed under sedation and local anesthesia. The operation is rarely performed under full general anesthesia. The reason is simply that sedation and local anesthesia are safe and effective for this procedure. Contrary to popular belief, a rhinoplasty is not a painful operation. Prior to the beginning of surgery, and after sedation has been given, the only discomfort felt is from several pinpricks for the introduction of the local anesthetic. The remainder of the procedure is not physically uncomfortable or psychologically traumatic. The operation itself takes up to an hour to perform, and is done entirely through the nostril opening. In most cases, no skin incisions are necessary.

In order to reduce or refine the nose, several steps are necessary. The bony upper portion of the nose must be reduced in size and refined in appearance. This requires breaking and resetting the bones, a procedure which is less formidable and far better tolerated than it sounds. The height, or hump in the profile, is then further altered by lowering the central portion of the nose. This is called the nasal septum, and it is made up of bone and cartilage. Care is taken at this point to produce the desired profile.

Changing the tip of the nose from bulbous to graceful-looking requires several steps. It is necessary to refashion four pieces of cartilage which support and shape the nasal tip. A number of highly technical steps are involved in each of these processes. At the end of the procedure, the nostrils are packed and the nose is covered with tape strips and a splint. The purpose is to allow the new nose to heal in the proper position.

AFTER THE OPERATION

Whether you recover in the hosital or at home, the first twenty-four hours will be much the same. Initially, you will be drowsy, experience some difficulty in breathing, have a headache, and generally be nonfunctional. You will be advised to rest in bed with your head elevated on several pillows. This serves to reduce swelling. Ice compresses may be used to inhibit swelling and discoloration around the eyes. After several hours, liquids can be taken by mouth. Breathing through the mouth becomes easier. Pain medications taken by mouth reduce discomfort, and you become more aware of your surroundings. There is a slight oozing of blood from the nostrils. This is normal and usually lasts through the first day or two.

After the first twenty-four hours, most patients are able to tolerate light diet and can care for themselves at home with little difficulty. Pain and discomfort are minimal. The majority of complaints are related to the nasal packing, which most surgeons remove between the first and fourth postoperative days. From the patient's point of view, removal of the packing is the highlight of the postoperative period, since this enables the patient to breathe through the nose again. Dressings and the splint, however, are not removed at this time.

After the first day or two of the postoperative period, the return to normal is rapid. Most patients have some discoloration and swelling around the eyes. For the first five days to a week, the nasal dressings and splint remain in place. Although the appearance of these is unsightly, few patients remain confined to their homes. Perhaps it is evidence of the acceptance of cosmetic surgery in our society that many postoperative rhinoplasty patients are not ashamed to be seen in public in this condition.

When the splint and the dressings are removed, the new you will be visible. Although not yet in their final form, the changes in the nose are dramatic. Most patients are advised to return to work and a normal life at this time. However, sports activities must be avoided for four to six weeks.

In the first few weeks, it is important to avoid forcefully blowing the nose. All manipulation of the nose is undesirable, and the patient is also advised to avoid heavy eyeglass frames. Some surgeons advise patients to tape their eyeglasses to the forehead to avoid any pressure on the nasal bones. Sneezing must be carried out with the mouth open. This allows air to rush out of the mouth, not the nose, and lessens the chance of nosebleed. Bending is acceptable as long as the head is not held below the level of the heart. This is important, since keeping the head in a dependent position may cause congestion and nosebleed. Along with the gradual return to normal activities comes progressive reduction of swelling about the nose. (When the splint is removed after surgery, the new nose is so much the focus of attention that the rather significant swelling around it is not noticed.)

Most patients visit the plastic surgeon about ten days after surgery to have a suture removed from inside the nose. This is the usual time for the question, "Is my nose still swollen?" By now, the patient has studied her new nose incessantly. She is aware of some thickness of the skin, and some loss of sharp contours, particularly at the top of the nose. This is absolutely normal. The swelling will recede rapidly over the next several weeks. But that is not the end of the story. The new nose continues to become thinner, more graceful and more refined until it achieves its final form at the end of about one year. Most of the changes are so gradual that the patient herself does not notice them. However, if photographs were taken at one month, three months, six months and twelve months postoperatively, significant change would be visible at each interval.

After approximately six weeks, the nose is no more likely to be damaged than an unoperated nose would be. Having had a rhinoplasty performed does not make the nose abnormal. If a baseball were to break your nose, this would be a significant but not earth-shaking event, just as it would be if your nose had never been operated on. During the first three to six months after surgery, however, patients who have undergone rhinoplasty should cover the nasal area with an effective sun-blocking agent during all periods of direct exposure to sunlight. The reason is simply that the skin has not yet returned to normal and will burn easily and swell extraordinarily. Some doctors apply the following common-sense rule: when all sensation returns to normal around the nose, then it is no longer necessary to take specific precautions against the sun. This is sound advice.

OPERATIONS TO BUILD A NOSE

Cosmetic nasal surgery includes several other procedures besides the standard "nose job." Among the candidates for these are individuals who, either from birth or accident, have absent or depressed nasal bones. Most often, a relatively normal nasal profile can be produced by inserting either carefully carved bone or hard silicone implants to fill the hollow areas on the nose. If bone is chosen, the usual donor site is the patient's own rib or hip bone. This adds significant discomfort and an element of fear to the procedure. Because of this, other approaches have been devised. The most successful of these is the use of carved silicone implants. This is less traumatic and more easily performed. The results are

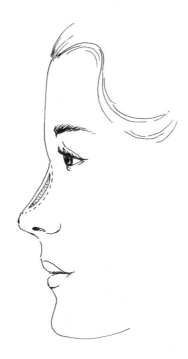

The addition of bone or synthetic material
to build up the nasal profile.

excellent cosmetically. The drawback is that in a large percentage of cases, over a period of time, the implants slip out of position, and re-operation or replacement may be necessary.

NOSTRIL REDUCTION

Another operation often performed alone or as part of a rhinoplasty is reduction of the nostrils. Individuals with large, flaring nostrils often wish them made less conspicuous. This can be done by means of a relatively invisible incision in the crease between the nostril and the cheek, through which the necessary amount of nostril is removed. A straighter, less flared look is the result.

Nostril reduction is often a necessary part of a rhinoplasty. When the bony structure of the nose is shortened, previously inconspicuous nostrils become flared and this sort of excision is necessary. It is a simple procedure which yields rich dividends in terms of the overall appearance of the nose.

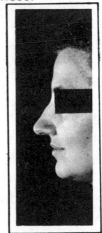 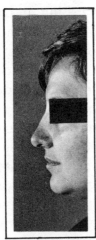

Pre-operative photo prior to reduction of nasal prominence.	After nasal reduction and nostril reduction.

CORRECTING A DEVIATED SEPTUM

In conjunction with cosmetic surgery of the nose, many patients request correction of a breathing obstruction caused by a deviated nasal septum. This is a condition in which the wall separating the two sides of the nose is deviated to one side, blocking the air passage in one nostril. It is usually most troublesome during allergy season, when the lining of the nose swells and the passage is occluded. It is not unusual to centralize the nasal septum at the time of rhinoplasty in order to allow easier breathing.

POSSIBLE COMPLICATIONS OF RHINOPLASTY

In addition to the problems associated with surgery in general, rhinoplasty has a few complications of its own. The most common is nosebleed. If this is to occur, it usually does so by the tenth postoperative day, but there is no hard-and-fast rule on this. Postoperative nosebleed is a disturbing and frightening occurrence, but in most cases it is easily dealt with by simple measures.

Infection is another possible complication. This is more serious, but it is exceedingly rare and can be dealt with effectively with modern antibiotics and surgical care.

The most common complaints after rhinoplasty are loss of sensation in the nasal tip and inability to smell. Fortunately, these are usually temporary problems which disappear over the first few postoperative months.

Although not truly a complication of surgery, the most common cause of patient complaint after rhinoplasty is an unsatisfactory cosmetic result. Assuming that the patient is realistic and the surgeon experienced, this problem is usually remediable. It is to be hoped that the days are past when any plastic surgeon will cavalierly remove too much cartilage and bone, leaving the patient with little more than nostrils. Most modern plastic surgeons, in fact, tend to lean toward the conservative side. In most cases of error today, therefore, the problem is that not enough has been removed, rather than too much. In such cases, minor adjustments several months after initial surgery are usually all that are necessary to produce a satisfactory result.

Nasal cosmetic surgery, as practiced today, offers the opportunity to achieve a dramatic change for the better. When it is combined with other techniques for balancing the facial features, the results can be remarkable. In general, just exchanging an unsightly feature for an unremarkable but normal-looking one is enough to change one's self-image as well as the outward appearance by which one is judged. The results of rhinoplasty often change the patient's entire outlook. It is the success of plastic surgeons in altering the perspective of the face by changing the nose, or nose and chin, that has made rhinoplasty such a readily accepted and sought-after operation. People who undergo this surgery are usually the plastic surgeon's most appreciative patients.

CHAPTER 6

BETTER LOOKING EARS

The term *cosmetic surgery of the ear* refers almost exclusively to otoplasty, a procedure which is often known as "pinning the ears back." Its purpose is to correct a situation in which the ear protrudes from the head and often looks very much like the handle of a teacup. The popularity of long hair for men and women alike has done a great deal to hide this deformity. However, styles change, and without surgical help, the ear will not.

In most cases, the cause of this deformity is absence of a fold in the ear which is referred to as the antihelix, or the antihelical fold. In the following photograph, you will see, in the abnormal ear, the absence of the back folding which keeps the ear close to the side of the head. The surgeon's task is to introduce the absent fold into the ear in order to more nearly approximate a normal situation. Absence of the antihelical fold is a characteristic often passed from generation to generation, and is more commonly found in some regions of the world than others. It is said that areas exist in the British Isles where this configuration is so common as to be considered normal.

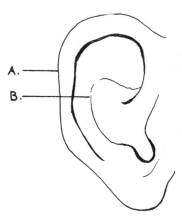

Normal ear A—Helix B—Anti-Helix

It is not unusual for only one ear to be involved, but most often the problem is evident in both ears.

In dealing with a child who has significantly unattractive protruding ears, several factors must be considered prior to surgery. It is essential, first of all, to wait until growth of the ear is almost complete before operating, so that later growth will not cause deformity. Nevertheless, it is desirable to perform the surgery before the child becomes aware of his deformity. Other children are adept at singling out such a child, and many can be merciless and unyielding when teasing their peers. This can

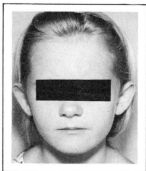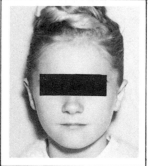

Child before and after otoplasty.

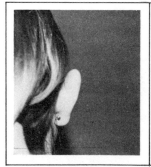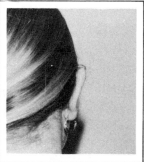

Posterior view
before otoplasty.

Posterior view
after otoplasty.

produce unhappy years for the child who is the butt of the "Dumbo" jokes.

Fortunately, the ear attains 85 to 90 percent of its full growth by the time a child is five years of age. Thus, it is possible to operate on a child at approximately four years of age, prior to his becoming the butt of classroom jokes but after his ear has reached nearly full growth. If it seems unlikely to you that a child's ears could achieve full growth by age five, just look around you. It is amazing the number of young children who appear to be "all ears."

Despite availability of this surgery, marginal or even severe cases are often hidden by long hair or altogether ignored. Ultimately, young adults arrive in the offices of plastic surgeons with stories of long-standing unhappiness due to this deformity. Happily, the operation can be performed at any age if only a few details are altered.

In the case of children, otoplasty is usually performed under general anesthesia, since it is difficult, if not impossible, to obtain the cooperation of a four-year-old child in the terrifying rituals of the operating room. Adults, on the other hand, are usually operated on in the office or outpatient operating suite under sedation and local anesthesia.

The operation is a relatively minor procedure causing little postoperative pain or disability. In fact, most patients complain only about the large dressing they must wear about the head for several days after surgery.

During the operation, a strip of skin is removed from behind the ear, following previously determined marks. To produce an antihelical fold or to increase the size of an existing one the cartilage must be altered. This can be done by cutting through the ear cartilage, by abrading the cartilage, or simply by bending the cartilage and suturing it firmly into its new position. The skin behind the ear is then carefully closed. Within weeks, there is little or no detectable sign that the surgery has taken place.

Postoperatively, the patient finds his ears carefully padded with cotton and gauze, and wrapped heavily with cotton and elastic bandages. The purpose of this is twofold: to apply pressure so as to discourage swelling and bleeding, and to hold the ear firmly in its new position. Depending on the surgical technique chosen, this bandage must remain in place from three to ten days. A shorter period of bandaging follows procedures in which the cartilage is actually incised. A longer period follows procedures in which the cartilage is bent and sutured.

After the bulky dressing has been removed and the area carefully cleansed, the patient must wear a nightcap or ski-type head band to bed every night for six weeks. This is to prevent him from accidentally disturbing the position of the ears during sleep.

Except for several days of minimal discomfort, the patient's only complaint is that the ear may be numb. It will also appear swollen for several weeks. These are normal postoperative symptoms which will disappear with time.

Otoplasty is simple and effective. Infection is the most serious complication but the incidence is exceedingly rare. The results of otoplasty are usually much appreciated by patient and parent alike.

CHAPTER 7

IF BALDNESS
IS A PROBLEM

There are a number of methods of disguising a bald pate. These vary from hairpieces to hair weaving to various semi-surgical procedures in which a hairpiece is sutured to the scalp. With the use of hair thickeners and various grooming agents, men have learned to get enormous mileage out of a few thin hairs. The popularity of the newer technique of hair transplantation seems to have coincided with the stylishness of longer hair for men. Whether one has stimulated the other is hard to determine, but many plastic surgeons, dermatologists and various other physicians are now inundated with requests for hair transplants.

Men go bald in a predictable pattern. In all cases other than those caused by illness, a ring of hair remains from ear to ear, even though the top of the scalp may be completely hairless. Hair transplantation makes use of the fact that this ring of hair-bearing scalp is permanent.

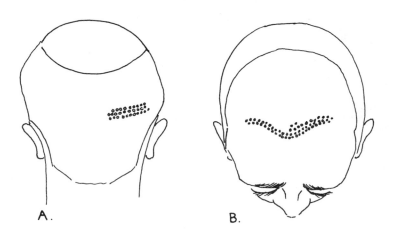

Hair plugs removed from donor site (A), and placed in bald area (B).

Small circles of hair, hair root and scalp 3.5 to 5 milli-meters in diameter are taken from this hair-bearing ring. Plugs of bald scalp of similar size are removed in a pre-determined pattern. The hair-bearing scalp plugs are then placed in the bald area. The donor site within the hair may or may not be sewn closed. The wounds heal, and the hair-bearing plugs retain the characteristics of the scalp from which they came. If all goes well, they will continue to produce hair indefinitely.

The hair transplant procedure must be carefully planned and mapped out in order to produce the most effective growth possible. Most experts strive for what appears to be a balding hairline, rather than attempting to create a teen-aged appearance. The result is not only more nat-ural looking, but easier to produce, and the mechanism is more difficult to detect. Even the best-performed and most successful hair transplants are not completely unde-tectable, however. Small bald areas remain between plugs, the quality of the hair may vary, and certain hair styles may be impossible to effect after surgery. Despite the drawbacks and limitations of hair plugs, they pro-duce normal, natural, permanent hair which most men find very much more acceptable than baldness or less natural-looking solutions to the problem.

A hair transplant operation is usually performed in the doctor's office operating suite. The patient is instructed to have no breakfast on the morning of the operation and is given sedation immediately prior to surgery. The pro-cedure is performed under local anesthesia, usually with the patient in a sitting position. The discomfort involved is simply that associated with the introduction of the local anesthetic. The procedure itself should be painless. After the proper number of plugs have been transplanted and all bleeding controlled, a large pressure dressing is placed around the head. This is removed in twenty-four to forty-eight hours. Then, gentle use of antiseptic shampoo may begin. At this point, the patient is instructed on scalp hygiene and may resume normal activities. Often there is a good deal of swelling about the forehead and eyes for a day or two after this operation. After surgery, the hair plugs are most frequently disguised by combing the remaining hair over the operated area.

A small stubble of hair is transplanted with the plugs to orient the new hair growth. After several weeks, however, these hairs are lost. The plugs remain bald for ten to twelve weeks, at which time new hair growth begins. The correction of baldness by hair plugs usually requires more than one operative session. Ancillary techniques such as strips of hair are also used when indicated.

Use of hair flaps is an even newer and more dramatic technique of treating baldness. In this operation, a two- to three-inch strip of hair-bearing scalp some six inches in length is used. The flap is based on an artery in front of the ear and is swung from the hair-bearing rim to the forehead region. The donor area is closed with sutures, and only a scar is noticeable. Usually a flap is developed from each side, and the two meet in the middle, forming a peak. Sometimes small hair strips or plugs are necessary to complete the procedure. The operation is performed in the hospital or office suite under general anesthesia. The procedure results in a full growth of permanent hair.

Among the problems associated with the hair flap procedure is the fact that there is a noticeable surgical scar

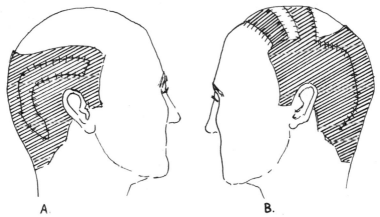

A.
B.

(A) Hair flap to be developed and rotated onto bald scalp.
(B) Flaps in place from both sides of scalp.
Line represents resultant in scar within hair.

just in front of the new hair. Moreover, the hair's direction of growth is toward the back, and therefore it does not help in disguising this scar. However, hair plugs may be used to camouflage the scar. Despite these drawbacks, most men are pleased with this very new method for developing a full and long-lasting head of hair. The procedure has gained great acceptance over the last two years, and appears destined to become a major method for the treatment of baldness.

CHAPTER 8

ALL ABOUT BREASTS

The size and shape of the female breasts have great psychosexual significance. In our society, breasts have become not only sexual objects but a yardstick used in the evaluation of a woman. They are also significant in a woman's evaluation of herself. We cannot assume that the breast is merely another functional body organ—a secretory gland and a skin appendage—although, in the strictest interpretation, it is little else.

To understand cosmetic surgery of the breast, one must first understand the breast. The bulk of the breast is composed of glandular tissue (breast gland), connective tissue and fat. It is covered with a skin brassiere and richly invested with blood vessels. The existence of a large network of sensory nerves throughout the breast accounts for its extreme sensitivity to pain, pressure and erotic stimuli. Each of the components of the breast is of great importance in maintaining its integrity. Therefore, in every surgical procedure performed on and about the breast, great care must be taken to avoid excessive disturbance of the delicate balance among these systems. A beautifully shaped breast in which the nerve supply has been obliterated becomes a graceful, but neuter, organ. If there is no longer a pathway for sensation and perception of erotic stimuli, the breast ceases to perform its sexual role. If the breast maintains its blood supply and nervous system but loses a large portion of the necessary skin coverage, it becomes a functional but unsightly organ. These unlikely and extreme examples serve to illustrate the point that an awareness of the anatomy and physiology of the organ is essential in devising and implementing surgical operations which minimize damage while producing the desired results.

The breast is attached to the chest wall almost as though it were an afterthought of nature. The exchange of nutrients and messages to the breast takes place through the nerves and blood vessels, which act as conduits between the internal and external environments. The hormonal stimulus for breast enlargement or lactation arrives via the blood vessels, and the end product, breast milk, is produced in the glandular substance of the breast and secreted through the ducts and to the outside via the nipple. There are no significant masses of voluntary muscles within the breast proper, which explains why exercise cannot increase breast size. There is no single major link from the breast to the body cavities. Therefore, the temporary or permanent removal of the breast from its natural position on the chest wall results in little or no functional change in the body as a whole.

Despite its size and weight, the breast is supported in its position on the chest wall by a thin veil of connective tissue fibers from the muscles of the chest wall, and principally by the holding ability of the skin brassiere that surrounds and covers it. There is no system of muscles, joints, tendons and ligaments to maintain the breast in position, as there is with other appendages such as the arm or the hand. It is therefore not in the least surprising that the high, firm breast of youth rapidly descends with maturity and sags woefully with increasing age.

The breast is very much like a weight suspended from an elastic band. For a while, the strength and elasticity of the band will suspend the weight satisfactorily. With loss of elasticity over time, the band will stretch, the weight will descend, and ultimately the shape and the relationship of the two objects will change beyond recognition. So it is with the breast.

With maturity, pregnancy and lactation, the breast increases in size. In the period after child bearing, there is a great loss of the substance of the breast, and an actual decrease in volume, as well as a loss of elasticity within the skin and suspensory tissue. One can easily understand how the shape, size and position of the breast rapidly change from the youthful ideal to the less desirable configuration of advancing age. Happily, the last twenty-five years have seen the design and perfection of surgical techniques which can compensate for many of these changes in a most remarkable and acceptable fashion.

Not every woman, of course, will experience sufficient deterioration of the breast to make her a candidate for plastic surgical repair. Most women find themselves, in maturity, with breasts that are somewhere between lovely young breasts and extensively aged ones. The changes may be significant, but tolerable. It is impossible to determine a specific point at which the normal and acceptable ends and the abnormal and unacceptable begin. This is a very personal matter which is predicated on a woman's self-image and on the relative value she places on her body, in general, and her breasts, in particular.

The first signs of aging in the breast are a shift of substance from the upper to the lower half of the breast, and a relative descent of the nipple. The usual yardstick for measuring breast descent is nipple position. As a rule of thumb, it is considered that in the erect body position the nipple should be approximately at the same level as the inframammary fold (the fold beneath the breast).

Other yardsticks used to determine change in breast height are the position of the nipple relative to the top of the sternum or breast bone, and relative to the mid-point of the clavicle or collar bone. Standards of what is normal in these respects vary with the height and size of the individual. The arms-over-head position is thought by many to represent the optimal nipple position, and some of the surgical procedures devised to rejuvenate and lift the breasts have been based on these measurements.

Pregnancies, breast feeding and weight change are responsible for many alterations in the volume of the breast and, with the aid of gravity, are responsible for great losses and shifts of breast substance, skin stretching, stretch marks and other changes. All of these are natural phenomena and cannot be prevented by brassieres, harnesses, lotions, potions or exercise. Weight reduction is perhaps the most distressing cause of these changes. Unfortunately, weight loss often begins in the least desirable places. Thinner faces and smaller breasts usually precede slim buttocks and a flat abdomen. This is a price many women pay to be fashionably thin.

CHAPTER 9

DO YOU WANT
LARGER BREASTS?

The simplest and most common of the cosmetic operations performed on the breast is augmentation mammoplasty or breast enlargement. The aim of this procedure is to augment, or enlarge, the already existing breast. It does not create a breast, but rather changes the physical appearance by adding substance from within, or more accurately, from behind. It is estimated that 150,000 breast augmentation operations are performed yearly in the United States.

The breast augmentation operation, as it is performed today, is somewhat more refined than it was some twenty years ago when it was first introduced in its modern form. Prior to the development of modern breast augmentation methods and materials, many bizarre, difficult and often unsuccessful procedures were devised to realize this goal. Even today, a plastic surgeon occasionally encounters patients who still have small, hard sponges imbedded in their breasts; breasts which are irregular and scarred because of unsuccessful attempts to enlarge them with abdominal or buttock fat; or breasts which are irregular, hard and often infected as a result of silicone injections. Fortunately, these crude techniques were never exceedingly popular. Today's procedures have been shown to be safe and effective, and hundreds of thousands of patients have benefited from them over the past two decades.

The augmentation procedure performed today is applicable to many circumstances, but it is most often considered in connection with the woman who simply desires fuller, larger breasts. Breast augmentation also serves well to replace breast substance lost because of aging, pregnancy or weight loss. It is useful in making ptotic (sagging) breasts seem less so by filling out the upper breast area. Essential to the procedure is the insertion of a prosthesis—a soft, nonreactive envelope containing a silicone gel or saline solution. Such prostheses are now produced by numerous companies.

The original envelope was a form of polymerized silicone produced by the Dow Corning Company and called Silastic®. The fact that Silastic is essentially nonreactive, soft, pliable and quite durable makes it as nearly ideal a substance as one could seek for this task. Other manufacturers produce similar material, and the properties and aims remain the same.

The soft envelope of the breast prosthesis is filled either with a saline (salt water) solution, which is similar to normal body fluids, or a silicone gel. Use of silicone gel in the prosthesis should not be confused with the unethical, illegal and dangerous use of liquid silicone injections into the breast substance. The silicone used to fill the breast prosthesis is unadulterated, and in a form which makes migration into the tissues most unlikely. The gel is of the same weight and density as breast tissue, and in over twenty years of use has proven safe and effective. Both saline-filled and silicone-gel-filled implants should be entirely undetectable after surgery. Both types are universally available, and each has its positive and negative features.

Under perfect conditions the results obtainable with both types of implant are natural, comfortable, and undetectable either visually or to the touch. The breast augmentation procedure is performed by placing the prosthesis between the breast and the chest muscle. In this manner, neither the chest cavity, the pectoral mus-

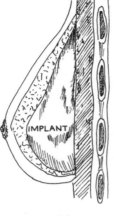

A cutaway view of the normal breast, the implant, and chest wall, as they would appear after surgery.

cles nor the breast itself is actually disturbed. An easily developed surgical pocket exists between the chest muscles and the breast, and it is into this nearly ready made pocket that the implant is generally inserted. (There are situations in which some surgeons favor placing the implant beneath the chest muscles. This is a somewhat more complex procedure, but it has been known to produce good results under certain circumstances.)
The incision through which the operation is performed is most often made at one of three sites.

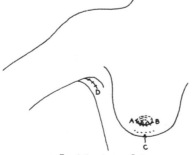

Incisions used in mammoplasty:
A-B Periareolar, C Inframammary, D Axillary.

THE INFRAMAMMARY INCISION

The most common type of incision is the inframammary (under the breast) incision. In this technique, an incision approximately two inches in length is made in the fold beneath the breast, and a pocket is developed behind the breast. An implant of the size previously agreed upon by surgeon and patient is then inserted behind the breast. Care is taken to place the implant in precisely the proper position for an aesthetically pleasing result. When the breast is of proper size and shape, the wound is closed with several layers of sutures beneath the skin. The patient may feel sure that she will have no difficulty with the wound and that the most insignificant scar possible will be produced by the surgery. A primary advantage of the inframammary technique is the fact that the scar will be hidden from view by the overhanging breast. After sufficient time elapses for the scar to mature, it will usually become difficult to see it at all.

THE PERIAREOLAR AND TRANSAREOLAR INCISIONS

The next most common site for the incision is what surgeons term the *periareolar* area. In this method, an incision is made in a semicircular or U-shaped fashion around the outside of the lower half of the pigmented portion of the nipple. (This is called the areola, and the incision is peri, or around, the areola.) The incision is carried through to the potential space between the breast and the muscles of the chest. The method differs from the inframammary approach primarily in the route taken to reach the pocket beneath the breast. Some surgeons favor cutting directly through the substance of the breast, in order to reach the desired plane. However, many others believe that this operation should be performed without disturbing the breast in any way. There are no long-term scientific studies available to show whether actually cutting through the breast tissue does any permanent damage, but it seems reasonable to avoid so bold a stroke whenever possible. It should be pointed out, however, that there are no reports of dysfunction, damage or complications as a result of this technique. After the implant is placed in the proper position, the wound is closed with care in a manner similar to the closing of an inframammary incision.

Use of the periareolar incision has several advantages and disadvantages. The incision is made at the point where the pigmented aerolar skin meets the normal, unpigmented breast skin. An incision in this area heals rapidly and with almost no detectable scar. An incision may be placed as a diameter across the nipple and areola. This results in little loss of sensation but necessitates incising the breast tissue. The areola and the nipple itself are the seat of the greatest majority of erotic and pressure sensations. The use of a periareolar incision often results in temporary and sometimes permanent loss or reduction of sensation in this area (the transareolar incision less so). There is a great deal of nerve supply to this area from every direction, so that total or major loss of sensation in a normal person is all but impossible. Additionally, most women report that over a period there is return of sensation to the area. It is impossible to determine objectively how much of this loss and recovery of sensation is real, and how much is subjective. These are factors, however, which should be considered by patient and doctor alike in choosing the proper incision prior to surgery.

THE AXILLARY INCISION

The third and least common method by which the same operation may be performed involves making an incision in the axilla. The axilla, or underarm, is a relatively distant and hidden site for the placement of the incision. The distance between the axilla and the breast, which aids in minimizing the visibility of the scar, also makes the operation less direct and therefore technically less desirable. Nonetheless, some surgeons believe that, on balance, this is often the proper route.

Despite variations in incision placement and surgical technique, type and size of implant, and implant position, most surgeons achieve excellent results using the methods with which they are most comfortable. Whatever the choices made, the postoperative breast should be natural in appearance and feel, and difficult to differentiate from a normal breast of similar size. The breast should flow and move and bounce normally, and there should be no visible edges or bulges. In fact, "only your plastic surgeon should know for sure."

OPERATING ROOMS AND ANESTHESIA

Breast augmentation can be performed in the hospital or the office operating suite. It can be performed under general anesthesia or with sedation and local anesthesia. Each method has its advocates among doctors and patients, but it is probably accurate to say that more and more surgery is being performed in the doctor's private office operating suite or in specially designed outpatient surgical centers. The majority of patients are up and about and able to perform light tasks shortly after surgery. What debilitation exists is minimal and very temporary.

The advantage of having the procedure performed under general anesthesia is complete amnesia regarding surgery. The drawback is the extensive period required for the body to metabolize totally and rid itself of the after-effects of the general anesthetic.

The positive side of sedation and local anesthesia is the fact that minimal confinement is necessary after surgery. Most patients are awake, alert, and can walk about freely after several hours. The drawback is that the patient must have absolute confidence in her doctor and must cooperate fully so that he may minimize medications and the discomforts of surgery.

On balance, it would seem that the patient undergoing the procedure with local anesthesia (usually a lidocaine-like substance) and sedation (usually tranquilizers) and pain medication does as well during surgery and recovers more rapidly than the patient having full general anesthesia.

There are, of course, a number of compromises between purely local and complete or general anesthesia. You should discuss these with your doctor prior to surgery.

CHOOSING THE RIGHT SIZE

The size of the breast prosthesis or implant to be used is determined by surgeon and patient together. Breast implants are produced and filled by cubic centimeters of volume either at the factory or by the surgeon. Each cubic centimeter (cc) represents an additional increment in size. A good rule of thumb is that 100 cc of increased size is the equivalent of one additional bra cup size.

The commonly quoted numerical chest measurement, or band size, is of little or no importance in describing breast size. For example, a woman who wears a size 38A brassiere has a large chest and small breasts. Chest size is of interest only insofar as the balance of the body as a whole is concerned. Breast augmentation will add to the chest measurement, but this is secondary, since our interest here is the breast itself.

How great an increase in breast size is desirable is a function of several elements. Of paramount importance are the wishes of the patient. The preferences of the patient's husband, boyfriend or other concerned individuals are much less significant. The patient is undergoing the surgery for herself, and must freely express her desires and needs, in order to attain the wished-for result. Within this framework there are several guidelines.

In the small-breasted but otherwise normal individual, the objective is to create a more acceptable feminine form. One must seek a balance between shoulder size, hip size and breast size, so that each is in proportion to the other. The grace of a well-proportioned body is the surgeon's goal.

The degree of enlargement possible is limited by the amount of skin available. The patient with almost no breast tissue and a thin frame will, while young, have very little lax or easily stretchable skin available about the breast. Therefore in this patient only a moderate increase in breast size is possible. If such patients wish to be larger still, a second procedure can be performed six months to a year later, after the skin and soft tissue about the chest have had an opportunity to stretch to an extent which will accommodate further increase in breast size.

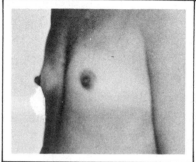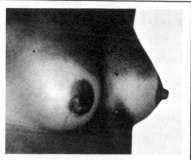

| Woman with very little natural breast tissue. | After augmentation to an appropriate size. The dark line below nipple is the inframammary scar. |

The woman who has smaller breasts than she desires, but breasts nonetheless, has greater latitude in the choice of breast size. It is not uncommon for such a woman to achieve an increase of one or more cup sizes. Thus, it is easier to change gracefully from a B cup to more than a C, than to go from less than an A cup to less than a B.

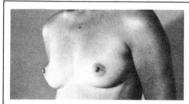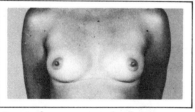

(A & B) Two preoperative views of a woman who lost substantial breast substance after pregnancy.

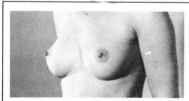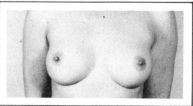

(A & B) Two post-operative views of same patient three months after surgery.

Another candidate for this surgery is the woman who, after childbirth, notices a marked diminution in her breast tissue without a corresponding decrease in breast skin. She notices an empty, hollow appearance in the upper portion of the breast, as well as various vertical stretch marks. For this woman, if she has not also been the victim of excessive sagging of the breast, augmentation produces very acceptable and often dramatic results. The implant size and shape are chosen so as to replace what has been lost. The aim of the operation is to fill out the empty skin at the upper portion of the breast and return a rounded, more voluptuous and less empty and hanging appearance to the breast.

Proper breast size is, of course, an individual and personal judgment. However, a good surgeon always stresses harmony. For example, a woman with a protuberant and somewhat flabby abdomen would do better to tighten her abdominal muscles and reduce her abdominal size rather than increase her breast size, while a woman with a thin and muscular abdomen and very small breasts might achieve proper balance by augmenting her breast size.

COMPLICATIONS

The results of breast augmentation surgery, in the hands of a qualified plastic surgeon, are almost always a delight to the patient. It is a well-controlled, well-tolerated operation, and the resulting full, graceful feminine breast is a reward for everyone concerned. However, problems may occur. In the manner in which the surgery is performed today, the incidence of major complications is very limited. They are certainly no more common than in similar forms of surgery upon external body structures.

The primary complication of breast augmentation surgery is a process called fibrous capsule formation. Although a great deal of research has been done on this problem, the precise mechanism for capsule formation, and therefore the means of controlling it, is still unknown. When the prosthesis is placed behind the breast, the body reacts as it would to any relatively inert foreign body. This reaction varies unpredictably from patient to patient, from operation to operation, and often from breast to breast. In everyone, a thin veil of scar-like capsule is formed around the implant. This is normal. In some patients, a thicker capsule is formed. When excessively thick, the implant is constricted by the capsule and forced into the shape of a ball, making it firm, sometimes uncomfortable and occasionally visible. The reaction of capsule formation is essentially a case of the body overdoing a good thing. The implant is not being rejected, nor is this a sign of infection.

These events have been estimated to take place in nearly 30 percent of cases, approximately half of whom exhibit firmness or discomfort. Thus, for almost 20 percent of patients who have undergone the operation, a corrective procedure may be necessary.

The most commonly performed and effective treatment for this problem is known as external capsulotomy. In this procedure, pressure is applied over the breast and capsule with enough force to crack the scar and allow the breast to become soft and natural again.

If this is unsuccessful, a surgical capsulotomy may be performed. This is a relatively minor procedure in which the incision is opened and the scar is released to allow expansion and softening of the implant.

In the overwhelming majority of cases of women who have undergone breast augmentation, the capsule formed is of normal thickness and does not produce any discernible symptoms. Of those in whom there is clinical evidence of capsule formation, the problem is most successfully dealt with by external capsulotomy, performed once or more than once until the problem is resolved. Rarely there is repeated capsule formation which cannot be controlled by manipulation, surgery or medication. In these cases, it is necessary to remove the implant entirely. If this should happen, the patient returns to her preoperative figure, with the possibility of trying again at a later date. Breast augmentation is a frequently performed, well-tolerated, and gratifying procedure which results in a minimum of significant complications. We have tried to provide a realistic and candid survey of the procedure. However, its benefits and problems should be dealt with

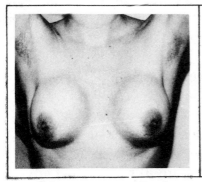
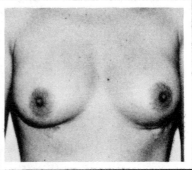

| An extreme example of fibrous capsule formation. The breasts are unnatural and firm. | After surgical expansion of the capsule and replacement of older type implants. |

on a considerably more personal level and in greater depth by each surgeon and patient. Whether aware of this information or not, many hundreds of thousands of patients—movie stars and mothers alike—have opted in favor of this procedure, and the overwhelming majority have been delighted with their new figures. However, a woman should know precisely what to expect and make an intelligent judgment based on fact, not fancy.

A BREAST AUGMENTATION CALENDAR

The following is a calendar of events that may be useful if you should decide to undergo breast augmentation.

1. Consultation and preoperative photographs.
2. Presurgical routine examination.
3. Surgery under local or general anesthesia.
4. Postoperative ambulation. Out of bed several hours after surgery.
5. Medication, food and liquids by mouth three to six hours after surgery.
6. Return home or spend the night in a convalescent facility or hospital room. The usual course following outpatient surgery is to return home four to six hours after surgery.
7. Medication to control pain and sleeping medications provided.
8. Antibiotics used at the discretion of the surgeon.
9. Twenty-four to forty-eight hours after surgery, bulky gauze and elastic bandages removed. From here after a soft bra may be worn. Many surgeons now advise "braless" weeks early in the course to aid in achieving a natural position and shape.
10. Forty-eight hours of limited activity and bed rest advised, head elevated at 30 degrees or on two pil-

lows. You must sleep on your back for two weeks, not your side or abdomen, as this can disturb the position of the implants.

11. Forty-eight hours after surgery, shower permitted using antiseptic soap.

12. On about the fourth postoperative day, gradual resumption of activities is permitted, excluding lifting of heavy objects, rapid reaching arms over the head, or driving an automobile.

13. At approximately the end of the first week, all skin stitches are removed and fine tape strips applied across the wound. These strips stay in place for approximately another week.

14. Four weeks after surgery, resume all normal activities and enjoy your new figure.

MAKING THE DECISION

Over the years, no increased incidence of breast cancer has been associated with this type of breast enlargement. Breast examinations are not hampered, mammography and breast feeding are possible, and changes in sensation about the breast are often minimal and temporary if they occur at all. These facts must be a part of your knowledge and discussed with your doctor when considering this surgery.

Prior to making a decision, however, it is vital to evaluate the reasons you wish to increase your breast size, decide whether or not such an increase is suitable to your figure, and digest all the information supplied here. If you decide to go ahead, you can look forward to a simple and easily tolerated operation and postoperative period, a rapid return to normal, and a pleasant and dramatic change in your appearance.

A BREAST LIFT

Breast lift, or mastopexy, is a term applied to the surgical elevation of a sagging breast. The problem of breast descent is essentially one of decreased elasticity of the skin and breast-supporting structures against the ever-increasing effects of gravity. As the breasts continue to descend, the skin which envelops them stretches. A less than aesthetically desirable appearance of the breasts results. The only solution to this problem is a surgical one. No amount of exercise, no breast potions or lotions, no creams or jellies and no miracle diet will help.

The concept of the breast lift operation is simple. The substance of the breast is not altered, but the skin envelope is trimmed and tightened. In this manner the breast mass and its nipple are moved up to a more attractive and youthful-looking site. The breast contour so created is generally excellent, and the hanging look is relieved.

Reducing the skin of the breast requires extensive skin incisions. (See illustration.) Periareolar as well as infra-

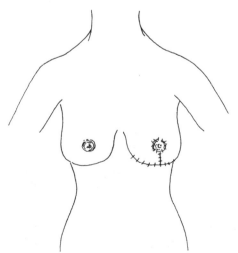

Location of scars following breast lift.

mammary incisions are generally made. A third, vertical incision joins the two. The nature of these incisions is such that scarring may vary from minimal to significant. In time, the incisions mature and become less noticeable. They do not disappear. Despite this drawback, most women who undergo this operation are more than pleased with the results. Here, as in all other surgery, it is critical to understand the cost in scarring, and to balance this carefully against the cosmetic improvement.

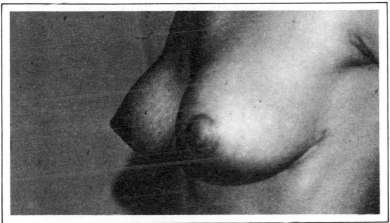

Result of breast lift three months after surgery to demonstrate position and extent of scars.

Many different complications can occur when this operation is performed by inexperienced or untrained surgeons. In the hands of experts, however, difficulties are considerably less frequent and less severe but they do occur. Most commonly, they include excessive scarring. Sometimes the breasts may appear asymmetrical (one larger than the other) or the nipples unequal in size or position. Fortunately, the majority of these problems can be corrected.

The photograph on page 99 is intended to demonstrate an average result, with average postoperative scarring from the breast lift procedure. It is possible to have significantly less noticeable postoperative scarring, or perhaps a more visible scar. The intent here is to provide a yardstick by which the prospective patient can more clearly understand what she is dealing with. It is, on the one hand, folly to believe that the breast lift can be performed without leaving any signs of operation. On the other hand, one must understand that in the overwhelming majority of cases the result is so favorable as to make the scarring acceptable.

CHAPTER 10

DO YOU WANT
SMALLER BREASTS?

Reduction mammoplasty, or breast reduction, is performed considerably more frequently than the breast lift. It is the most formidable of the breast operations, and is carried out under general anesthesia.

In appropriately selected patients, breast reduction yields gratifying results. The oversized bosom, whether simply very large or frankly enormous, is often a source of interest and amusement to men, but is more likely to be a 10-pound albatross about the neck of the woman so endowed. Comfort in motion, grace in dress, and self-confidence are impossible in the face of massively oversized breasts.

The cause of the oversized bosom, referred to medically as gigantomastia or virginal breast hypertrophy or macromastia, is difficult to pinpoint. True virginal breast hypertrophy is a condition in which the pituitary gland produces an abnormal amount of the hormone that stimulates breast growth. Under these circumstances even repeated surgery, short of total mastectomy, will not control the enormous overgrowth of breast tissue. Recently, however, medical means have been developed which can interrupt this process.

The majority of women who see plastic surgeons with the problem of overly large breasts have no clearly apparent hormonal problem. The overwhelming majority of patients with very large breasts have no postoperative regrowth, and the breast reduction procedure entirely corrects the problem.

The breast reduction operation has been designed to produce graceful, well-shaped breasts of a size proportional to the patient's body. Excessively large pigmented areolae can also be reduced by this procedure. Variations of this operation have been popularized internationally through the work of Strombeck in Sweden and Pitanguay in Brazil, as well as that of many American plastic surgeons. The basic approach is similar.

Breast substance must be removed in addition to skin. An attempt is made to preserve the sensory and erectile functions of the nipple, but the primary objective is to reduce the mass of the breast. It is not uncommon for as much as two to three pounds of tissue to be taken from each breast.

Of the various remarkably similar techniques available for breast reduction, the great majority fall into one of two major categories.

NIPPLE GRAFTING TECHNIQUE

In this group are operations in which the nipple and areola are first removed from their position on the breast, and then the surgical breast reduction and recontouring are carried out. On completion of this stage of the operation, the proper nipple position is determined and the nipple-areola complex is replaced as a skin graft. This technique has the advantage of allowing creation of excellent breast contours, and the drawback of markedly reduced nipple sensitivity and capability of erection. For these reasons, operations in which the nipple is removed and reapplied as a skin graft are reserved either for patients with the most enormous breasts, or for those in the older age group who are willing to sustain any loss of sensation so long as breast size is adequately reduced.

PEDICLE TECHNIQUES

In the second category are procedures in which the nipple remains attached to the remainder of the breast as though on a slender stalk. In surgical jargon, this is called a pedicle. In this technique continuity is retained between breast and nipple, and there is less significant reduction in sensation or erectile capability. Breast contouring is limited by the need to retain the nipple on the pedicle, which cannot be stretched beyond certain limits. Therefore, although it ensures an aesthetically acceptable result, the pedicle technique restricts the volume of breast tissue which can be removed. This operation is the type of reduction mammoplasty most commonly performed, and is suitable for reduction of moderately large breasts in younger women.

RESULTS OF BREAST REDUCTION SURGERY

The following photographs reveal average results of standard breast reduction procedures. Clearly visible is the single greatest drawback of this operation: the scarring which may result from the extensive surgical incisions. The pattern of incisions is the same as that described for breast lift, and the pattern of healing is similar. After a sufficient period has elapsed for maturation, the scars usually assume the color of the surrounding tissues and become significantly less noticeable. However, there is a tendency after breast reduction for scars to stretch.

From the time of surgery, approximately one year is necessary for the breasts to achieve their final appearance. However, the shape is nearly normal from the start, and the resulting appearance is a great deal more attractive than the huge and unsightly breasts for which the patient sought the help of her plastic surgeon.

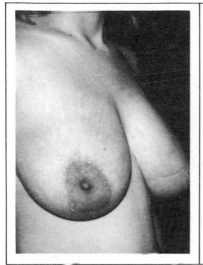
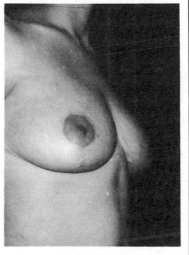

Pre-operative condition. Massive breast hypertrophy.

One year after breast reduction. Scars have faded and shape is good.

COMPLICATIONS

Complications associated with this surgery include the possibility of excessive or unsightly scarring, the possibility of loss of small amounts of breast skin near the suture lines which eventually heal, and unequal breast size or nipple position. Some degree of loss of sensitivity may also occur. These problems do not occur in every case but, when they do appear, are dealt with surgically and usually present no permanent problem.

The reduction of the overly large breast is a difficult task. Many surgeons feel it proper to inform the patient that following the operation there is the possibility of returning to the minor surgery operating room some six months later to touch up small areas of scarring or deal with other minor problems which may require attention. It is important for the patient to know this prior to surgery so that she will not become alarmed when informed of this at some later date. Meanwhile, she may enjoy her new shape and freedom from the heavy weights which were dragging her down both mentally and physically. It is likely that no further surgery will be necessary, but if such is needed, it should be treated as the second step of the surgery which the patient most anxiously sought.

Women about to undergo breast reduction should know that whatever procedure is chosen, they should not expect to be able to breast-feed following surgery. In the case of nipple grafting, there is total severing of all the breast ducts, and therefore breast milk may be produced but not delivered, causing engorged and cystic breasts. In the nipple pedicle type of operation, many ducts persist but many are cut as well, and lactation again may cause engorgement and cyst formation within the breast. If breast-feeding is of critical importance to the patient, the operation must be postponed until after the child-bearing years. Most women contemplating this surgery are so distraught with their present state, that they see inability to breast-feed as inconsequential.

POSTOPERATIVE CARE

Breast reduction surgery, like breast lift surgery, is performed under general anesthesia. Following surgery, for a period of up to a week, the breasts are firmly bandaged with bulky gauze and elastic dressings. In the first two weeks after surgery, a series of doctor's office visits are made in which the sutures are removed in stages and tape strips applied in their place.

For the first week after surgery, medication is necessary to control the small amount of pain and discomfort from the surgery. Antibiotics are not routinely used, and following the removal of dressings the patient is permitted to shower.

After fourteen days, normal activity is gradually resumed. At four to six weeks all activities, including sports, may be resumed. The patient will find that over the first six months to a year breast shape will continue to change, and change for the better. Prior to surgery, the effects of gravity are taken into account, and the change seen after surgery is part of the plan. Wearing a bra becomes optional for the first time in the patient's memory.

EQUALIZATION OF ASYMMETRICAL BREASTS

If one were to examine each and every woman very critically, it would be exceedingly rare to find perfectly matched breasts. In most women, there is some variation in size between breasts. Usually, however, the differences are small and not readily noticeable.

The following illustration shows a woman with perfectly normal breasts. Unfortunately, they are markedly different in size. A one-sided breast reduction was carried out in order to produce the result seen below.

In the case just illustrated, the patient chose to have the larger breast reduced. In other cases, the patient may choose to have the smaller breast made larger. In still other cases, one breast is considerably too large and the other very much too small. The proper course would be to enlarge the small breast and reduce the other.

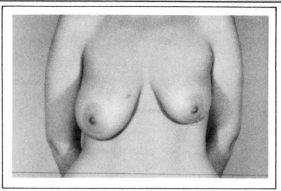

Breast assymetry.

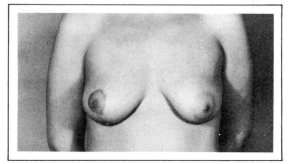

Six months after correction of assymetry
by reduction of right breast.

CHAPTER 11

RECONSTRUCTION
AFTER MASTECTOMY

Each year, for the last twenty-five years, approximately 80,000 American women have undergone mastectomy for treatment of cancer of the breast. Radical mastectomy includes the removal of the breast and the pectoral muscles of the chest. In many centers, less-than-radical mastectomies are routinely performed. Whatever the procedure, the aim is removal of every trace of malignancy, and total cure. Ninety percent of women who have adequate surgery, with no evidence of spread at the time of surgery, are cured of the disease. However, the patient is left with a significant deformity, which is not easily dealt with.

Traditionally, the general surgeon treating breast cancer has counseled the patient not to worry about losing the breast. She is advised to thank God for being alive. Perhaps there is a good deal of wisdom in this, but in our society, unfortunately, too much emphasis is placed on the female breast for such a matter-of-fact attitude to be adopted. The woman is forced to disguise her deformity and call up all her psychological reserves to deal with the problem. The gravity of the situation varies among individuals, but it is always painful and unhappy.

Over the last several years, through the techniques explored and developed for augmentation mammoplasty, plastic surgeons have become increasingly able to reconstruct the breast lost to cancer. Compared to a natural, normal breast, the breast produced by postmastectomy reconstruction is less than perfect. Compared to absence of the breast after mastectomy, however, the reconstructed breast is nothing short of a miracle.

A breast reconstruction operation is usually performed at about six months after mastectomy. It is felt that this period is necessary for the effects of the surgery to settle down, and to be certain there are no local recurrences of disease. During this time, and often even prior to the cancer surgery, the patient is introduced to the plastic surgeon and to the possibility of breast reconstruction. The simple act of meeting the plastic surgeon at this time often makes the breast removal less traumatic and the situation more hopeful for the patient.

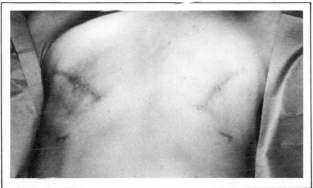

Bilateral mastectomy patient before reconstruction period. (*Courtesy Dr. R.H. Guthrie, Jr.*)

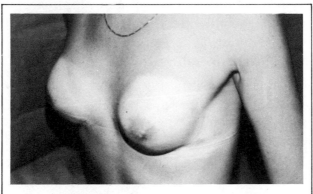

After bilateral breast reconstruction by
techniques described.
(*Courtesy Dr. R.H. Guthrie, Jr.*)

AN OPERATION IN STAGES

The breast reconstruction operation is performed in stages. The first consists of surgery under general anesthesia, at which time the skin overlying the chest wall is elevated. A secondary incision, or sometimes the original surgical incision, is used. It is necessary to develop a healthy skin flap, with underlying fat padding. When this stage has been completed, a breast prosthesis, usually one filled with silicone gel, is placed in the pocket in precisely the same manner as for breast enlargement. The wound is closed with several layers of sutures. It is most often left unbandaged so that the flap of skin may be observed in the early postoperative period. Antibiotics are usually administered. Pain medication is necessary for several days. Activities are limited for a week or two, and are gradually resumed as healing progresses.

Several months are allowed to elapse before the second stage of surgery. This is directed either at further enlarging the size of the breast or, if necessary, at repositioning the implant. An areola and nipple are also created at the second operation. This operation can be carried out under general or local anesthesia, in the hospital or office operating suite.

In addition to reconstructing the breast lost to cancer, several other procedures are possible. If the remaining natural breast is large, it is sometimes necessary to reduce its size in order to achieve a symmetrical appearance. This is necessary since the reconstructed breast, no matter how elegantly created, is limited in its size and its ability to take on the characteristics of a sagging mature breast.

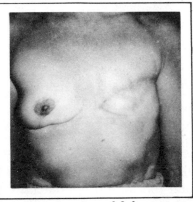

Before reconstruction of left mastectomy,
and right subcutaneous mastectomy.

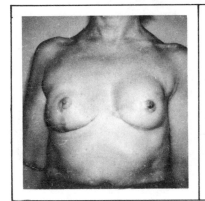
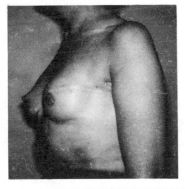

After left breast reconstruction, small implant
inserted into right breast.

The reconstructed breast is a marked improvement over
the condition in which one breast has been removed. A
relatively normal shape can be developed. The nipple is
created either of pigmented vaginal lining or from excess areola of the other breast. Additional methods have
been developed which allow the new nipple a normal
central projection. The entire procedure is being per-

formed with increasing frequency. The resulting reconstruction has become more elegant, and the final appearance now more closely approximates the normal breast. Other, more complex procedures are also available to make reconstruction possible when local problems make surgery as described unlikely.

COMPLICATIONS

Due to a number of factors, the complications of postmastectomy breast reconstruction are legion. The skin flap under which the implant is placed is thin, and often has a less-than-perfect blood supply. Therefore swelling, discoloration, infection and occasional skin breakdown may occur. A collection of fluid under the flap may persist for weeks or months. The size, shape, position and even the appearance of the nipple may not be wholly acceptable. Unfortunately, this is the state of the art. However, it has been very rare for a woman who has undergone this procedure not to be pleased with the results. Although the operation is not perfect, the preoperative and postoperative conditions are worlds apart.

CHAPTER 12

SUBCUTANEOUS
MASTECTOMY

ᢓᢓᢓ

Subcutaneous mastectomy is a procedure in which an attempt is made to shell out the substance of the breast through a series of skin incisions. The breast is reconstructed, immediately or at a later date, with a prosthesis. The purpose of this operation is to reduce or eliminate the possibility of breast cancer. Several facts concerning this operation make it quite controversial among surgeons. To begin with, it is impossible to remove 100 percent of breast tissue by this technique. The areas of particular difficulty are in and about the nipple and sometimes the upper outside tail of the breast. Even if 95 percent of the breast is removed, cancer may develop in the remaining 5 percent. (Incidence of breast cancer in women with small breasts is no less than incidence in women with large breasts.) Some physicians dispute this, reasoning that 95 percent of the possibility of breast cancer has been eliminated. Nonetheless, breast tissue remains.

The results of subcutaneous mastectomy are almost uniformly less than perfect. Difficulties include hard breasts with irregular surfaces, skin breakdown, and asymmetry between breasts. Despite these not uncommon complications, many women who have undergone this operation are thoroughly satisfied with the results and are relieved to believe they have reduced the chance of incurring breast cancer.

This operation is not offered to, nor intended for, all women. It was devised as a method of treating several situations. Among these is that of the woman who has undergone multiple breast biopsies and has a strong family history of carcinoma of the breast. Other candidates have been said to include women with cancer

phobia and women in whom certain low-grade neo-
plasms of the breast have been discovered. This procedure is essentially therapeutic, and should be discussed
more fully with your surgeon or plastic surgeon before
you decide that it is for you.

CHAPTER 13

REDUCING AND
TIGHTENING THE ABDOMEN

The face and breasts are not the only areas of the body subject to the insults of age and time. The entire body is constantly fighting the law of gravity. Whatever is up must eventually come down. Fortunately, indignities thus visited upon the body can be dealt with as successfully as those affecting the face.

The concept of cosmetic surgery of the body is probably a great deal less familiar to you than that of face lift, eyelid surgery or nasal surgery. Over the years, however, plastic surgeons have become adept at dealing with unsightly or aging portions of the body as well as of the face and neck. The idea of body sculpturing began with the breast and has grown to include the abdomen, buttocks, thighs, and even the arms, legs and hands.

Abdominoplasty is one of the medical terms used to describe an operation in which excess, wrinkled or stretched abdominal skin is retailored and surgically smoothed. Nearly a dozen techniques fall into this category: Each operation is designed to remove excess skin, or skin and fat.

The average individual with a large belly is not a candidate for this surgery. Here, diet and exercise, vigorously applied in a disciplined manner, are all that are necessary. They should do wonders to melt away excess flesh and tone up the abdominal muscles. The change happens slowly, and patience is necessary. The results, however, can be nothing short of spectacular.

Surgical treatment is reserved for special situations. Those patients who have been massively overweight, and have had the self-discipline to win the fight against obesity are prime candidates. These people often find the abdominal skin does not shrink back to normal size.

They are left with a great apron of unsightly hanging skin as a reward for their dedication and hard work. Theirs is the classic case in which abdominoplasty performs wonders of transformation. Others who will benefit from this surgery include women who have not recovered their shape after pregnancy.

The results of this surgery vary directly with the need for it. Individuals with the most obviously loose and redundant flesh which will not respond to further diet or exercise have the most significant improvement from this surgery. The flaccid abdomen after pregnancy benefits as well. The not-so-loose abdomen, with a few stretch marks and a bit of excess fat, will achieve a certain new grace of form, but a magic transformation is neither necessary nor possible.

Abdominoplasty is not a substitute for exercise. It is an adjunct. It should be resorted to only after diet and exercise have done all they can.

Patients who have undergone abdominoplasty are usually delighted with the results. They must be informed prior to surgery that certain scars must unavoidably be created. If this is not fully explained, or if the patient has unrealistic aspirations, disappointment will be the inevitable result.

An important aspect of the art of plastic surgery lies in placing scars where they will be least conspicuous. Prior to abdominoplasty, the patient is asked to put on the briefest of underpants. The lines of this garment are traced onto the skin. In most cases, it is possible to contain the incisions from abdominoplasty within the confines of these lines. The scars themselves are usually placed in or near the groin creases at the top of each thigh and across the pubic hair.

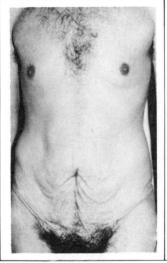 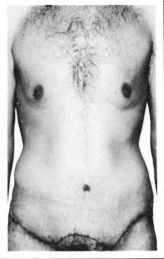

| Before surgery— much loose skin on abdomen. | Immediately after surgery abdomen is smooth and firm. Scars will soon fade to normal skin color. |

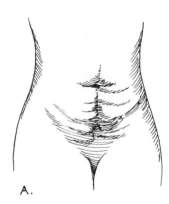 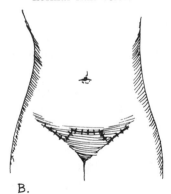

A.   B.

Artist's illustration of the photos above,
showing location of scars.

Abdominoplasty requires elevation of all the skin and fat from the abdominal wall, from the pubic area to the chest. The belly button is surgically preserved so that it may be replaced in its new position. If there is weakness between the abdominal muscles, it is repaired at the time of surgery.

The operation is performed with the patient's hips flexed, and the skin of the abdomen is then pulled tight to the level of the incision. The excess is trimmed away, and the new, taut abdomen is sutured into its final form. When a heavy dressing or plaster mold has been applied over the abdomen, the operation is complete.

Although abdominoplasty can effectively remove nearly all the excess tissue on the anterior (front) part of the abdomen, it cannot remove the excess on the flanks, back or buttocks. Separate procedures are required. Some surgeons perform these procedures together, but most believe it best to divide the work into two or more sessions.

The complications possible with abdominoplasty are those of surgery in general. Bleeding, infection or breakdown of wounds can occasionally occur in this or any other surgical procedure. Most patients find the operation uncomplicated and rewarding.

If you are contemplating abdominoplasty, you can expect something like the following sequence of events.

Surgery is usually performed in the hospital. Prior to surgery, you will be placed on a liquid diet. Enemas and laxatives will be given to reduce the need for bowel movement in the early postoperative period. Although this will be unpleasant the night before surgery, you will be glad for it the first few days after the operation. For several days prior to surgery, you will probably be asked to refrain from the use of aspirin, and to shower using an antibacterial agent. Antibiotics may or may not be administered prior to surgery.

The operation will be performed under general anesthesia. After surgery you will awake in the recovery room, usually with your knees and hips flexed and your head and shoulders raised. You will be asked to breathe deeply and cough. This will be most unpleasant, but it serves to prevent postoperative lung complications. There will be some pain and discomfort for the first few days. Often the most annoying complaint is the inability to urinate on the evening after surgery. Catheterization may be necessary. (This means draining the bladder with a tube.) After twenty-four to forty-eight hours you will be out of bed and walking to the bathroom.

From here on, things become relatively easy. After the first few days, the drains will be removed from the skin and dressings will be changed. For a while your abdomen will feel so tight that you will walk hunched over. This is normal, and gradually you will become able to assume a normal position. After two or three weeks, all sutures are removed. Tape may be applied to the wounds for various periods to prevent stretching of the scars. Normal activities, including exercise and sex, are resumed between four and six weeks after surgery.

CHAPTER 14

The buttock lift is another type of body sculpture which is frequently performed today. The patients who benefit most are those with buttocks which are excessively large or overhanging and out of proportion to the rest of the anatomy. Others who are good candidates include individuals who have lost a great deal of weight and have empty hanging skin over the buttocks.

The buttock is a combination of muscle mass, fat and skin. The operation removes skin and fat. It does not change the large muscular buttock. The incision is placed inconspicuously, in the crease below the buttock. This is marked with the patient erect. The patient is anesthetized and placed in face-down position. A large wedge of skin and fat is removed. The amount depends on the quantity of excess present. There are limits to what can be done with this procedure, but usually a significant portion of the excess buttock can be removed.

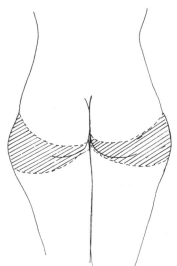

Area of fat and skin to be removed from
buttocks and outer thighs.

The scar extends from the inside portion of the thigh, beneath the buttock to the outside portion of the thigh. Some of this outside portion may be visible beneath or above the briefest of bikinis. The majority of the scars are easily hidden in slightly more modest garments.

The change in shape should be dramatic. The biggest complaint following this surgery is, "I can't sit down." It is ten days to two weeks before the patient is permitted to sit fully in a chair. Most patients say that this is a small price to pay for a sleek new shape.

FLANK RESECTION

When people have lost a great deal of weight, there is often excess skin on the flanks. This is not removed in either the buttock or the abdominal repair. It is necessary to make additional incisions to remove this overhang. The incisions should be placed as inconspicuously as possible, but each case is individual and must be dealt with on that basis. The combination of abdominal lipectomy or abdominoplasty, buttock resection and flank resection can totally transform an irregular, sloppy and flabby appearance to a tight and more appealing look.

In these procedures it is not unusual for small irregularities to occur at the edge of each incision. This is due to the huge amount of tissue being removed. These "dog-ears" are easily dealt with at a later date. Additionally, there may be spreading and overgrowth of the scars somewhere along the incision. This, too, can be dealt with later. Many surgeons feel that a period of three to six months should be allowed to elapse before contemplating touch-up surgery.

HIP AND THIGH SURGERY

There are a number of well-known operations for reducing bulk on the outside of the thighs and flabbiness of the inside of the thighs. The procedure for removing the fat on the hip or outside thigh is directed at what is called a riding breeches deformity. This term is applied because of the similarity between the patient's appearance and the configuration of the classic riding trousers. In medical language, this is known as trochanteric lipodystrophy, which means an abnormal amount of fat on the hip.

Surgery to correct riding breeches deformity is performed in the hospital under general anesthesia. Incisions begin in the outermost portion of the fold beneath

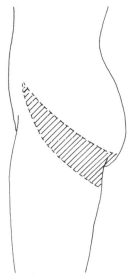

Area of fat and skin to be removed at the outside of the thighs and buttocks.

the buttock and move up toward the hip bone. The majority of the incision is hidden by any garment larger than a bikini. The scars are not of the fine hairline variety, but they do eventually assume the color of the surrounding skin.

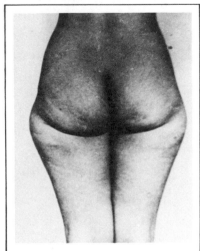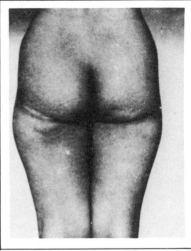

Before and after correction of riding breeches deformity.

This procedure is performed in order to change the shape of the torso dramatically. It is not meant to correct minor deformities. The scarring from this operation though not awful, is significant enough to restrict it to those people in whom the change in shape would be well worth the resulting scar. The inner aspect of the thighs is often the site of flabby excess fat. This can be removed, and the skin tightened, by an incision in the groin crease at the top of the thigh. The change in shape can be most pleasant and rewarding. More extensive deformities or hanging skin sometimes require the use of a small vertical incision as well. In this surgery, there are often problems related to the scars. The vertical scar, although important for achieving good contours, remains visible. Because of the tightness of the repair, the groin scars are sometimes pulled from the groin and may become visible at the top of the thigh. All these scars gradually blend with the surrounding tissue and are the price paid for the change in shape. Both the riding breeches and the inner thigh operations are usually performed in the hospital under general anesthesia. Recovery generally entails several days of bed rest and a gradual return to normal activities over a period of two to three weeks.

GUARDING AGAINST BLOOD CLOTS

In all surgery performed on the abdomen, buttocks or thighs, one precaution is observed above all others: the need to guard against the formation of blood clots in the legs. In order to protect against this, patients routinely wear compressive dressings or elastic stockings over the calf. Exercise is begun early, and patients are allowed out of bed within the first forty-eight hours after surgery. These measures, as well as others, including certain medications, greatly reduce the incidence of thrombophlebitis (blood clots) after all varieties of surgery.

Body sculpturing leaves scars. It also produces changes in shape which are often impossible to achieve by any other means. When diet, exercise and other methods have failed you must decide how serious these defects are to you, before you can determine whether you really want to have them corrected surgically. If you are realistic, informed and motivated, this surgery can solve a multitude of problems and greatly improve your appearance.

CHAPTER 15

BEAUTIFYING
THE ARMS AND HANDS

The present-day emphasis on youth and beauty is all-encompassing. Very often a person has aged gracefully except for loosely hanging skin on the upper arms. In other instances, a person may lose weight, generally tone up and make significant strides in personal improvement, only to find the effect spoiled by loose, old, skin of the arms and hands. Previously, the answer to the problem was a long-sleeved garment, and conspicuous attempts to make the hands inconspicuous. With today's abbreviated fashions, it has become more and more impossible to mask this problem. The mature person still enjoys an active outdoor life and wants to dress appropriately for this. Plastic surgeons have thus been faced with the problem of correcting upper arms and hands in individuals who are otherwise well satisfied with their appearance. Progress has been made, but the results are not perfect or fully accepted.

The most common method of combating hanging fat and skin in the upper arm is a direct attack. In this method the surgeon evaluates the problem and estimates the amount of excess fat to be removed. An incision is made in the undersurface of the arm, usually in a repeating W-shaped pattern. The purpose of this type of incision is to prevent the scar from shrinking and causing a post-operative deformity. The operation works well in that the excess is dramatically removed. The problems are related to the scar which is created.

Even when the scar matures to take on the characteristics of the surrounding tissue, it is still not invisible. However, most patients who have had this surgery would rather have a scar on the inside of the arm than flabby, old-looking upper arms.

The surgery can be performed in the hospital or outpatient suite, under local or general anesthesia. It is relatively minor in relation to other plastic surgery procedures.

Recovery time is short. Sutures are removed in seven to ten days, and tape strips are applied across the wound for a somewhat longer period. Activities are restricted for several weeks. Pain and discomfort are minimal.

Some excess skin is necessary for the elbow joint to fold and unfold properly. However, wrinkled, relaxed excess skin about the elbow is often a concern to older individuals. A number of relatively minor procedures are performed which remove an ellipse of skin above the elbow area. This eliminates some of the inelastic hanging skin. The surgeon avoids placing a scar directly over the elbow joint. This procedure is not intended to produce dramatic results, and very few people are candidates for it.

The wrinkled elderly hand is a problem that has annoyed both doctor and patient since plastic surgery began to make advances in combating the ravages of age in other areas. A patient looking at her wrinkled, pigmented hands may lose her enthusiasm for the excellent surgical rejuvenation that has been done in other parts of her body. Innumerable methods have been devised to deal with the problem. Very few have gained acceptance.

There are essentially two methods of tightening the skin on the hands. One is to pull the skin upward to the crease of the wrist or downward toward the knuckles. The excess skin may be excised in a zigzag manner in the interspaces of the fingers. This technique avoids later scar contracture. The other method combines removal at the wrist with an incision on the small finger side of the back of the hand. This results in an L-shaped incision through which excess skin is removed. These procedures have been described on many occasions but are infrequently indicated and infrequently performed.

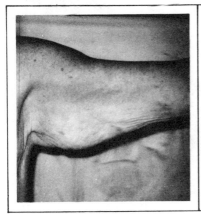

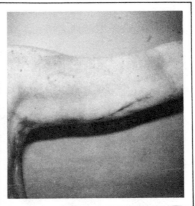

Excess skin and fat of upper arm.

Two months after surgical removal of excess. Scars will later assume color of surrounding skin, but never disappear completely.

CHAPTER 16

SELECTING A
PLASTIC SURGEON

Developing the ability to select competent physicians is an integral part of becoming an educated and intelligent consumer of medical care. When you are placing your physical and mental well-being in the hands of an individual, it is important to know as much about him as possible. In medicine, as in all other matters in which choices are made, it is important to understand the ground rules and to learn to use them in locating those professionals who can be of greatest assistance to you.

According to the licensing laws of most states, any licensed physician, regardless of training and experience, may declare himself a plastic surgeon. For that matter, any licensed physician may limit his practice and declare himself a practitioner of any specialty he may select. This is his legal right, long supported by a significant portion of the medical establishment and government.

In today's supertrained society, however, the finest and most rigidly prepared specialists are readily available. It therefore seems unfortunate that the public should be misled into thinking that a self-proclaimed specialist has the blessing of the medical community and the good of the public at heart. To understand the full significance of this, imagine that your family doctor, as competent, warm and wonderful as he may be, one day decides to take down his "General Medicine" shingle and replace it with one saying, "Practice Limited to Neurosurgery." Although this might well be perfectly legal, it would not assure you of the highest quality neurosurgical care.

We live in an age when medical and scientific progress is unfolding at such an enormously rapid pace that it is difficult for one individual to keep track of, let alone master, the developments in even a small area of medicine. Residency training programs were devised in order to provide the most diligently trained, competent and up-to-date practitioners of the specialties. Most prorams have expanded, and competency examinations have been developed in an attempt to establish and maintain the highest possible standards. These are standards by which the various specialists judge themselves and their peers, and these have little or nothing to do with the legalities and politics of who can do what in medicine.

The present governing board for plastic surgery is an organization called the American Board of Plastic Surgery, located in St. Louis, Missouri. It is this Board, incorporated in 1937, which seeks to standardize the training of plastic and reconstructive surgeons at the highest level possible. The purpose is to enable the public to rest assured in the knowledge that their surgeons have at least undergone the procedures deemed necessary to train a plastic surgeon, and that they are eligible to take the Board certifying examination and/or have already passed this examination and been certified by the Board.

Does this mean that because your surgeon finished medical school, and spent a year as an intern, four years as a general surgery resident and two years as a plastic surgery resident, he is guaranteed to produce the best possible result on your upcoming face lift? Not at all. What it means is that such a plastic surgeon has been properly trained according to the body governing his specialty, has proven himself sufficiently acquainted with the techniques of plastic surgery, and has sufficient experience in the practice of plastic surgery to offer you what we hope is an acceptable level of expertise. It does not suggest that a minimally trained surgeon with a great technical hand and artistic mind cannot produce fine examples of creative plastic surgery. It merely states that, all else being equal, a Board certified plastic surgeon has undergone what is considered proper training for a plastic surgeon in order to minimize the risks of deficiency. It is probably fair to say that a great majority of people think of this individual when the term *plastic surgeon* is used, and therefore perhaps some differentiation should be made among practitioners of plastic surgery to avoid misleading the public.

Ear, nose and throat specialists, or otolaryngolotists, or, as some prefer to be known, facial plastic surgeons, are another well-established specialty whose members do a considerable amount of good work in plastic surgery. This specialty encompasses a large number of surgeons who are, as a rule, well trained in performing procedures about the head and neck. Over the years, a great number of ear, nose and throat specialists have performed increasing volumes of plastic surgery. In fact, many of the early leaders of the plastic surgery community were members of this specialty group. Many of the training programs in otolaryngology include exposure to plastic surgery, and there is a good deal of healthy overlap between the specialties. As a rule, ear, nose and throat plastic surgeons consider themselves primarily facial plastic surgeons and rarely perform sculpturing and reconstruction of the body or breast surgery.

Here, there is no black or white, right or wrong. To put it simply, one should know the training, the Board certification or eligibility and the hospital affiliations of a surgeon. Being aware of, and carefully measuring, these criteria should help reduce the element of chance when selecting a plastic surgeon. In addition to hospital and teaching activities, the observation of a job well done and the recommendation of respected members of the medical community are of paramount importance in obtaining the best possible plastic surgical care.

In most cases, however, choosing a plastic surgeon is somewhat different from selecting any other physician. In cosmetic surgery, all procedures are elective. The patient is neither ill nor under extreme pressure to have the procedure performed immediately. He may therefore pick and choose among surgeons. There is time enough to ask the proper questions of the people involved, in order to attempt to ensure a healthy doctor-patient relationship and a rewarding surgical result.

At last count, there were 1,712 plastic surgeons certified by the American Board of Plastic Surgery. These surgeons are listed by city and state in the Appendix of this book. In addition, there are several hundred men and women in training to become plastic surgeons. The number of plastic surgeons has more than doubled in the last ten years, and the demand for cosmetic surgery has more than outstripped this increase. There are now very few areas in the United States that do not count a plastic surgeon among their physicians. This is a testament to a new public awareness and acceptance of cosmetic surgery, and to the fact that this art and science has been developed to a point at which the results justify this enormous popularity.

There are many societies, educational and otherwise, to which the majority of plastic surgeons belong. Perhaps the most useful of these, from the consumer's point of view, is the American Society of Plastic and Reconstructive Surgeons, Inc. This organization is located at 29 East Madison Street, Suite 807, Chicago, Illinoiis 60602 (telephone 312–641-0593). Besides disseminating well-thought-out information, the Society will also supply you with a list of qualified plastic surgeons in your area. Doctors' names are chosen on a random and rotating basis, so that preference for one surgeon over another is avoided. In most cases, the three names provided you by the Society will be among those listed in the Appendix of this book.

Many libraries own reference copies of the *Directory of Medical Specialists*. In this volume, all Board certified physicians are invited to list their training and appointments, which are then arranged by specialty and area for easy reference. The *Directory of Medical Specialists* does not list those who have completed their training but not yet completed certifying examinations. This is unfortunate since in medicine generally a large number of young, well-trained but as yet uncertified specialists are in the forefront of their fields, and plastic surgery is no exception.

We hope that this short course in how to pick your plastic surgeon will be useful. After you have secured the names of the plastic surgeons in whom you are interested, and "checked them out," it will be time to meet your surgeon, discuss your problem, ask the questions you feel are important, get to know him and give him an opportunity to know you. The idea is not, however, to test the surgeon, and you will be doing yourself a great disservice if you ask either unnecessary or excessively technical questions. It is of little importance to you whether your plastic surgeon will suture with silk or nylon material, and you will be wasting valuable time necessary for surgeon and patient to understand one another. The aim, after all, is to enable the plastic surgeon to become aware of your desires and to balance these against his evaluation of your needs. He must also evaluate you as a patient and a person.

Among the key factors for success in plastic surgery are a realistic and motivated patient, and an honest and interested surgeon. Once a relationship between two such individuals has been satisfactorily established, another step has been taken toward your ultimate goal.

Now you have made the decision, "This is my doctor." Once this determination has been made and is based, hopefully, on sound judgment as well as intuition, you must have full faith in the skills, honesty and integrity of your surgeon. Your doctor, being human, responds well in such an atmosphere, and you will have done your best to establish the proper circumstances under which to maximize your chances for complete satisfaction.

ADVERTISING IN MEDICINE

The last year or two has found the medical profession involved in enormous turmoil over the concept of advertising. In several states, particularly California and New York, direct action of licensing bodies has made it known that, within guidelines, physician advertising is felt to serve the public good. This is an opinion shared by a number of Federal regulatory agencies. They believe restricting professionals from advertising is in restraint of trade and a disservice to the public. They reason that allowing physicians to advertise under guidelines which prohibit false claims and comparisons allows the public to become aware of professional services which would otherwise be unknown to them. It is felt that advertising facilities and fees would spur competition among professionals, to the benefit of the public. Whether this is true is debatable. Nevertheless, medical advertising has begun and it will, in all likelihood, continue.

What the individual seeking cosmetic surgery must keep in mind is that choosing a surgeon purely on the basis of advertising is similar to entering a busy intersection blindfolded. You may arrive safely, but this is not the best way to cross the street. Advertising may help you understand what is available, but your research should not end there. You must learn as much about your surgeon as you can. This is not to imply that superbly talented and dedicated physicians will not advertise their services, but merely that untrained and even inept physicians may advertise as well. Other criteria must be applied to increase your chances for the best possible result. The simplest of these is a full knowledge of your surgeon.

CHAPTER 17

THE COST OF BEAUTY

Fees charged for cosmetic plastic surgery vary from community to community. The following chart offers the approximate range of fees throughout the United States. There will certainly be exceptions at both ends of the scale, but the relative costs of various procedures should be evident. The figures quoted represent surgeons' fees for the operative procedures and postoperative care. *They do not include hospital costs, operating room charges or consultation fees.*

The usual consultation fee varies from $25 to $75, and is paid at the time of the visit. If surgery is performed, the consultation fee is sometimes deducted from the surgical fee. If this is the case, it is usually so stated. Consultations vary in length. Their purpose is to answer questions and to examine and evaluate the patient.

Increasingly, insurance carriers are unwilling to cover expenses incurred at the hospital in connection with cosmetic surgery. A great many carriers also totally exclude reimbursement for surgeons' fees related to cosmetic surgery. This situation places financial stress on the patient. The insurance companies are specifically excluding physician and hospital costs related to plastic surgery in many new policies. However, they also attempt to evaluate fairly cases in which there are medical indications or other pressing needs for surgery.

Because the cost of forty-eight hours of hospital care and two hours in the operating room can be more than $1,000, alternatives have been sought. The most acceptable solution has been development of the private surgical suite or ambulatory surgical center, which take advantage of the fact that the majority of plastic surgery operations can be safely performed outside the hospital.

Most of these procedures are purely external in nature, and are not very debilitating. It has been found, through experience, that patients recover successfully and comfortably at home or in an aftercare facility. The close proximity of the surgeon to the patient in the all-important early postoperative hours has been found to be an additional favorable factor in the development of outpatient surgery. Under these circumstances, the fee charged to the patient for use of the facilities varies from $50 to $250, depending on the procedure performed. Realizing that there are enormous savings to all concerned, insurance companies may begin to reimburse for this fee. The savings to the patient can be significant.

Whether a procedure is done on an in-hospital or an out-patient basis, the surgeon's fees remain the same.

Rhinoplasty (nasal reshaping)..$1000-$3000
Blepharoplasty (eyelids)............$1000-$2500
Brow lift ....$ 750-$1500
Temporal lift...............................$1000-$2500
Full face lift ....$1500-$4000
Full face lift and eyelids...........$2000-$5000
Chin augmentation......................$ 500-$1500
Chin reduction ....$1000-$3000
Otoplasty (ear reduction or
   pin back)..................................$ 750-$2500
Chemical face peel......................$ 500-$1500 Depending on area treated
Facial Dermabrasion ....$ 500-$1500 Depending on area treated
Breast augmentation ....$1000-$3000
Breast lift....................................$1500-$3500
Breast reduction ....$1500-$4000
Abdominoplasty ....$2000-$4000

Thigh and hip reduction............$2000-$4000
Buttock reduction.......................$1500-$3500
Hair transplants ....$ 15-$ 25 per plug
Hair flaps...................................$2000-$4000

So many other procedures and combinations of procedures are done that it is impossible to list them all here. The fees above represent the range throughout the country for the services listed. Fees are generally based on the operative and postoperative time spent on each procedure. The value of this time varies from surgeon to surgeon, and from place to place. Higher fees do not guarantee better surgeons. Lower fees are not necessarily a bargain.

WHY PAYMENT IN ADVANCE?

Plastic surgeons, as a rule, require full payment of their fees prior to surgery. (This is not the procedure followed by most other medical specialists.) The reason is that cosmetic surgery is an elective, planned and non-emergency procedure, in which the patient is not required by physical need to complete the surgery within a given time. Therefore, the rate of postponement and cancellation of surgery has been found to be inordinately high compared with the rate in other specialties. This, combined with the fact that the busy plastic surgeon must plan his surgical schedule weeks if not months in advance, makes it necessary for him to be certain that the schedule will not be upset when the patient has accepted a last-minute social invitation. If surgical fees have been prepaid, the likelihood of unnecessary disruptions such as those are minimized. Additionally, a high percentage of a plastic surgeon's patients may be from outside his local community. This makes billing postoperatively an extraordinary chore. Finally, human nature being what it is, some surgeons believe that an individual is more likely to be pleased with the result of a procedure for which he has already paid, than with the result of one for which he is about to be billed. Whatever the rationale, prepayment is the rule in cosmetic surgery, and it apparently has functioned well over the years.

IF YOU CANNOT AFFORD THE SURGEON'S FEES

What should do if you cannot afford the fees of a private plastic surgeon? First, a word of caution. Cosmetic surgery is not the sort of purchase in which one should seek a bargain. Here, one must be concerned with quality and only secondarily with cost. If you hear about a surgeon whose fees are remarkably below those of qualified surgeons in the same community, you owe it to yourself to check carefully his credentials, his reputation and his work. This is not to say that plastic surgeons do not, as a rule, significantly lower their fees or work free when the situation warrants it. Generally, in fact, plastic surgeons in private practice donate a portion of their time to plastic surgery clinics, where they supervise and assist residents in training. Through these clinics cosmetic surgery at nominal fees is available to the public.

Nearly every major university and every major hospital has a plastic surgery clinic. Here the surgery is performed by resident plastic surgeons who are experienced, in varying degrees, with the procedures within the scope of plastic surgery, and perform them through the clinic according to their level of ability.

In addition, a number of organizations have been formed in various areas of the country through which plastic surgeons donate their services on a rotating basis and perform surgery without charge.

CHAPTER 18

ON BEING REALISTIC

As you may remember from the beginning of this book, our goal was to guide you through the possibilities and pitfalls of cosmetic plastic surgery. We asked the question, "Is it for you?" We hope that after reading this volume you are closer to the answer.

As you continue thinking about plastic surgery, you should keep in mind the fact that in surgery and nature there are no absolutes. General knowledge of a surgeon's work and his academic credentials is not a guarantee. Additionally, be cautioned that no one is perfect. You were not perfect prior to surgery, your surgeon is not perfect, and, try as he may, he cannot produce absolute perfection.

If you combine the facts we have given you with some common sense, we believe that you will be delighted with the improvement cosmetic surgery can provide, and the lift it can give to your self-esteem.

Good luck.

APPENDIX

The following section is produced as a service to the readers of this book. Listed by state and city are individuals certified by the American Board of Plastic Surgery as of 1977. Additional information concerning these surgeons can be obtained at your library in the *Directory of Medical Specialists.* We cannot guarantee that names haven't been inadvertently excluded.

The fact that an individual is certified by the American Board of Plastic Surgery does not guarantee good results, and many specialists trained in other disciplines may also produce excellent surgical results. Being on this list means only that an individual has completed a prescribed training program, and has passed the examination given for certification by the American Board of Plastic Surgery.

ALABAMA

BIRMINGHAM • HOWE, ROBERT E., M.D. • MARZONI, FRANCIS A., M.D. • NICKELL, WILLIAM B., M.D. • OLIVER, ROBERT J., M.D. • PITTS, WILLIAM J., M.D. • ROBINSON, O. GORDON, M.D. • SHERLOCK, EUGENE C., M.D. • STREICHER, ROBERT E., M.D. **HUNTSVILLE** • BURLISON, PAT E., M.D. • WALKER, GEORGE R., JR., M.D. **MOBILE** • CROSBY, JOHN F., JR., M.D. • GREEN, BYRON E., JR., M.D. • GREEN, JAMES W., M.D. **MONTGOMERY** • CONNELLY, DAVID M., M.D. • NOBLIN, WILLIAM E., M.D.

ALASKA

ANCHORAGE • ADDINGTON, DONALD B., M.D. • MALLIN, ROBERT E., M.D. **FAIRBANKS** • WENNEN, WILLIAM W., M.D. **KETCHIKAN** • CARLSON, GARY E., M.D.

ARIZONA

MESA • BUNCHMAN, HERBERT H., II, M.D. • WISNER, HARRY K., M.D. **PHOENIX** • BAINS JERRY W., M.D. • BARTON, MORRIS, JR., M.D. • BULL, JOHN C., JR., M.D. • CALLISON, JAMES R., M.D. • CARROLL, DANIEL B., M.D. • DODENHOFF, THEODORE G., M.D. • FRIEDLAND, JACK A., M.D. • HUDAK, THOMAS M., M.D. • JOHNSON, CLARE W., M.D. • LAWRENCE, HOWARD C., M.D. • MacCOLLUM, MAXWELL S., M.D. • McGREGOR, ROBERT J., M.D. • NORTON, ROBERT E. G., M.D. • PETERSON, REX A., M.D. • ROSENBERG, SIDNEY A., M.D. • SUDJARITRUKSE, SUCHART, M.D. • WOHL, RICHARD H., M.D. **SCOTTSDALE** • HAIT, GLEN, M.D. • SIMONS, JOHN H., M.D. **TUBAC** • NATTINGER, JOHN K., M.D. **TUCSON** • BURKHARDT, BOYD R., M.D. • FLEISHMAN, PHILIP, M.D. • MADDEN, JOHN W., M.D. • PEACOCK, ERLE E., M.D. • SCHNUR, PAUL LEO, M.D. • TOFIELD, JOSHUA J., M.D. • WHITACRE, WENDELL B., M.D.

ARKANSAS

LITTLE ROCK • ALLEN, THOMAS H., M.D. • HAYES, HARRY J., JR., M.D. • POPE, NORTON A., M.D. • STUCKEY, JAMES G., M.D. **ST. JOE** • STUTEVILLE, O. H., M.D.

CALIFORNIA

ALHAMBRA • SEIF, ALI A., M.D. **ALTADENA** • HATCH, MERTON D., M.D. **ANAHEIM** • KLEIN, ANDREW W., M.D. **ARCADIA** • COSTARELLA, ROBERT J., M.D. **BAKERSFIELD** • SARMICANIC, SCHAUL, M.D. • SCHMIDT, GERHARD H., M.D. • SCHWARTZ, ADOLF, M.D. **BERKELEY** • BRANDFIELD, ROBERT T., M.D. • YAHR, JAMES H., M.D. **BEVERLY HILLS** • AIACHE, ADRIEN, M.D. • BIRCOLL, MELVYN J., M.D. • FARNSWORTH, DIANA V., M.D. • FLYNN, MICHAEL P., M.D. • GURDIN, MICHAEL, M.D. • KERN, FRANK B., M.D. • LAKE, STEPHEN, M.D. • LEAF, NORMAN, M.D. • SARNAT, BERNARD G., M.D. • SOKOL, ANTHONY B., M.D. • WAGNER, KURT J., M.D. **BURBANK** • McDOWELL, ALLYN J., M.D. • RAMSDEN, CHARLES H., M.D. • WHITLOW, DENNIS R., M.D. **BURLINGAME** • GRADINGER, GILBERT P., M.D. • KAUFFMAN, RAYMOND R., M.D. **CANOGA PARK** • SENGLEMEN, ROBERT P., M.D. **CARMEL** • McLEAN, DONALD H., M.D. **CARMICHAEL** • RYBKA, F. JAMES, M.D. • VAN ROOYAN, KIRK W., M.D. **CASTRO VALLEY** • IVERSON, RONALD E., M.D. • KOHN, ELEANOR MARIE, M.D. • LOEFFLER, ROBERT A., M.D. **CHICO** • CREECH, BREVATOR J., M.D. • MANGUS, DONALD J., M.D. • MORGAN, L. RICHARD, M.D. **CHULA VISTA** • UMANSKY, CHARLES, M.D. **CONCORD** • MURPHY, STEPHEN M., M.D. • RANSDELL, ALLEN M., M.D. • TOLLETH, HALE R., M.D. **DALY CITY** • MALONEY, SEAN, M.D. **DANVILLE** • SIEGFRIED, GEORGE E., M.D. **DAVIS** • BAKER, KENNETH D., M.D. **DOWNEY** • BRODY, GARRY S., M.D. • KOONIN, ALFRED J., M.D. • MARSCHALL, FRANZ E., M.D. • REED, CLARENCE C., M.D. • WILSON, LIBBY F., M.D. **EL TORO** • ROHRER, PAUL A., M.D. **ENCINO** • GOLDBERG, HERBERT M., M.D. • GROSSMAN, A. RICHARD, M.D. • MARSHALL, FRANZ E., M.D. • ROSENTHAL, SHELDON A. E., M.D. • ZIMMERMAN, RICHARD W., M.D. **FONTANA CITY** • IMPROTA, ROBERT S., M.D. **FOUNTAIN VALLEY** • PAUL, MALCOLM D., M.D. **FREMONT** • ZANDI, IRAJ D., M.D. **FRESNO** • GEIS, JOHN R., M.D. • GOSHGARIAN, GEORGE G., M.D. • RYSKAMP, JAMES J., JR., M.D. • SILSBY, JOHN J., M.D. • TAKAYAMA, NORIO, M.D. • TUR, JUAN JOSE, M.D. • WILDE, NORBERT JOHN, M.D. **FULLERTON** • MABIE, PAUL D., M.D. • STERLING, HARLEY E., M.D. **GLENDALE** • BELLINGER, CREIGHTON G., M.D. • KROSNOFF, JOHN A., JR., M.D. • PERRY, ALLAN W., M.D. **GREENBREA** • DAKIN, RICHARD L., M.D. • JAQUA, RICHARD A., M.D. • MANIS, JOHN R., M.D. • MINAMI, ROLAND T., M.D. **HAYWARD** • EPSTEIN, LEONARD I., M.D. • TUERK, DANIEL B., M.D. **HUNTINGTON BEACH** • KAMPER, MICHAEL J., M.D. **LA JOLLA** • LEWIS, CARSON M., M.D. • MAJURE, O. LAMAR, M.D. • SINGER, ROBERT, M.D. **LAKEWOOD** • CHUNG, BOK S., M.D. **LA MESA** • HOYT, C. JAY, M.D. • SMITH, DAN SULLIVAN, M.D. **LOMA LINDA** • HARRIS, CURTIS N., M.D. • SLAYBACK, JOHN B., M.D. • ZIRKLE, THOMAS J., M.D. **LONG BEACH** • BLOOM, MYRON J., M.D. • CUNNINGHAM, DANIEL S., M.D. • KELLEHER, ROBERT C., M.D. • KLINGBEIL, JEROME R., M.D. • KRUGMAN, MARK E., M.D. • WOOD, DAVID L., M.D. **LOS ALTOS** • JOBE, RICHARD P., M.D. • NICHOLSON, JOHN L., M.D. • **LOS ANGELES** • ASHLEY, FRANKLIN L., M.D. • BIRNBAUM, LAWRENCE M., M.D. • CLIFFORD, CHARLES A., M.D. • CORWIN, THEODORE R., M.D. • DeSHAZO, BILLY W., M.D. • FRILECK, STANLEY P., M.D. • GOIN, JOHN M., M.D. • GRIFFITHS, CADVAN O., JR., M.D. • HANSEN, WILMER C., M.D. • HARDIN, BRYON, M.D. • KAWAMOTO, HENRY K., JR., M.D. • KIRIANOFF, T. GREGORY, M.D. • LESAVOY, MALCOLM A., M.D. • MILLER, TIMOTHY A., M.D. • OLSEN, JOHN A., M.D. • PEGRAM, MAX W., M.D. • RHODES, ROBERT D., III, M.D. • SCHREINER, E. OLIN, M.D. • SEIFERT, LAWRENCE N., M.D. • SEMEL, GEORGE H., M.D. • SHEEN, JACK H., M.D. • TAGAVI, BIJAN, M.D. • TEARSTON, GARY M., M.D. • THOMPSON, DENNIS P., M.D. • WILLIAMS, JOHN E., M.D. • WORTON, EUGENE W., M.D. • ZAREM, HARVEY A., M.D. **LOS GATOS** • TABARI, KUROS, M.D. **LYNWOOD** • NOBLE, JAMES H., M.D. **MISSION VIEJO** • ZLATNIK, DONALD F., M.D.

150

MODESTO • ANDERSON, D. GORDON, M.D. **MONTEREY** • HOOKER, THEODORE C., M.D. • WILCOX, REX G., M.D. **MONTE RIO** • HADLEY, RUSSEL C., M.D. **MOUNTAIN VIEW** • ROSENBERG, HOWARD L., M.D. **NAPA** • GRISEZ, JAMES LOUIS, M.D. **NEWPORT BEACH** • BERNBECK, VOLKERT J., M.D. • CHONG, J. KENNETH, M.D. • GRAZER, FREDERICK M., M.D. • HEINRICHS, HARVEY L., M.D. • LUHAN, JORGE E., M.D. **NORTHRIDGE** • NEMETZ, JOSEPH C., M.D. **NOVATO** • YOSOWITZ, PHILIP, M.D. **OAK-LAND** • CARSON, WILLIAM E., JR., M.D. • GRUBER, RONALD P., M.D. • HOSKINS, H. DEAN, M.D. • JONES, HYZER W., M.D. • KAHN, RICHARD A., M.D. • PATTON, DOUGLAS S., M.D. • PATTON, HENRY S., M.D. • SCHNEIDER, PAUL J., M.D. • SCRIMSHAW, GEO. C., M.D. • SHEPARD, RICHARD A., M.D. **OCEANSIDE** • KELLETT, CYRIL F., JR., M.D. **ORANGE** • CASEY, ROBERT E., M.D. • FURNAS, DAVID W., M.D. • WANGSANUTR, LIKHIT, M.D. **PALM DESERT** • ROWLAND, WILLARD D., M.D. **PALM SPRINGS** • KAPLAN, BRUCE A., M.D. • TIPTON, JOHN B., M.D. **PALO ALTO** • APFELBERG, DAVID B., M.D. • BERNER, ROBERT E., M.D. • COMMONS, GEORGE W., M.D. • HENTZ, VINCENT R., M.D. • KAPLAN, ERNEST N., M.D. • KEOSHIAN, LEO A., M.D. • LASH, HARVEY, M.D. • MASER, MORTON R., M.D. **PASADENA** • MORGAN, STANLEY C., M.D. • WEBSTER, GEORGE V., M.D. **POMONA** • CALAYCAY, LIGORIO A., JR., M.D. **RANCHO PALOS VERDES** • CHHABRA, AJAIB S., M.D. **REDDING** • SHADDISH, WILLIAM R., M.D. **RED-LANDS** • YOUNG, FORREST, M.D. **REDONDO BEACH** • CHAO, WEN YING, M.D. **REDWOOD CITY** • MILLER, FRED W., M.D. **RICHMOND** • LEE, HOWARD, M.D. • LUEDERS, HAROLD W., M.D. • SHAPIRO, ROBERT L., M.D. **RIVERSIDE** • CORBET, PAUL A., M.D. • TUCKER, ANDREW L., M.D. **ROSS** • GOLDSTEIN, MARCY A., M.D. **SACRA-MENTO** • BRUNER, JACK G., M.D. • BURKE, LEON O., M.D. • COCKE, WILLIAM M., M.D. • COOK, ORRIN S., M.D. • FAGGELLA, ROBERT M., M.D. • GONG, KINMAN, M.D. • HAMILL, JAMES P., M.D. • HAUSE, DONALD P., M.D. • OSBORN, JOHN M., M.D. • PRATT, FREDERICK E., M.D. • RICHARD, E. FREDERICK, M.D. **SALINAS** • KELLOGG, DONALD R., M.D. **SAN BERNARDINO** • ANDERSON, DENNIS K., M.D. **SAN DIEGO** • CRAWFORD, JAMES, M.D. • DEFIEBRE, BRUCE K., JR., M.D. • ESCAJEDA, RICHARD M., M.D. • FISHER, JACK C., M.D. • GLASS, LEONARD W., M.D. • GLEASON, MATTHEW C., M.D. • KRUGGEL, JOHN LOUIS, M.D. • MANCHESTER, GARY H., M.D. • MOORE, LAWRENCE T., M.D. • NOBEL, GARY L., M.D. • PICKERING, PAUL P., M.D. • RUDOLPH, ROSS, M.D. • VECCHIONE, THOMAS R., M.D. **SAN FRANCISCO** • BLACKFIELD, H. M., M.D. • BOLLINGER, KARL J., M.D. • BROWN, E. C., M.D. • BROWNSTEIN, MICHAEL L., M.D. • BYRNES, WILLIAM P., M.D. • CAPOZZI, ANGELO, M.D. • EMERY, JOHN EDWARD, M.D. • FALCES, EDWARD, M.D. • FRIEDENTHAL, ROGER P., M.D. • FRIEDMAN, GARY D., M.D. • GORNEY, MARK, M.D. • GREENBERG, ROGER L., M.D. • HARRIES, THOMAS P., M.D. • HOVEY, LESLIE M., M.D. • KAUTH, JAMES H., M.D. • McGREGOR, MAR W., M.D. • MOGLEN, LESLIE J., M.D. • MORRIS, WILLIAM J., M.D. • OUSTERHOUT, DOUGLAS K., M.D. • OWSLEY, JOHN Q., M.D. • PENNISI, VINCENT R., M.D. • RISTOW, BRUNO, M.D. • STEISS, CHARLES F., M.D. • TOMLINSON, FRED B., M.D. • WEINER, MICHAEL D., M.D. **SAN JOSE** • AVAKOFF, JOSEPH C., M.D. • BROCK, CLAYTON E., M.D. • BERK, LEO H., M.D. • ELLENBERG, ALEXANDER H., M.D. • GUALTIERI, ANTHONY C., M.D. • LUCID, MORGAN L., M.D. • MILLS, ROBERT L., M.D. • PARDOE, RUSSEL, M.D. • SOUTHER, SHERMAN G., M.D. • STANGER, JAY V., M.D. **SAN LUIS OBISPO** • JORGEN-SEN, JERREN E., M.D. • KING, DALE W., M.D. **SAN MATEO** • BUNCKE, HARRY J., JR., M.D. • GONZALEZ, RICHARD I., M.D. • THUSS, CHARLES J., M.D. **SANTA ANA** • CAVON, JOSEPH F., M.D. • CONNELL, BRUCE FOWLER, M.D. • CRAWFORD, HUGH H., M.D. • MINNER, ROBERT T., M.D. • STRONG, JOHN O., M.D. **SANTA BARBARA** • CHAPPLE, JOHN G., M.D. • DIETRICH, SANFORD R., M.D. • NAGEL, G. PETER, M.D. • STEPHENSON, KATHRYN L., M.D. **SANTA CRUZ** • LOWE, RODNEY S., M.D. • PLETSCH, MARIE E., M.D. **SANTA MONICA** • AMONIC, ROBERT S., M.D. • CHIZEN, JOHN H., M.D. • CLAVIN, HAROLD D., M.D. • DAVIS, GERALD N., M.D. • EDWARDS, BENJAMIN F., M.D. • WILMS, FRED J., M.D. • WOOTON, D. GARETH, M.D. **SANTA ROSA** • BUCHHOLZ, ROBERT B., M.D. • MELLERSTIG, KENT E., M.D. • TRUCKER, ALBERT L., M.D. **SOUTH LAKE TAHOE** • FOSTER, LAWRENCE H., M.D. **STANFORD** • BRENT, BURTON, M.D. • LAUB, DONALD R., M.D. • VISTNES, LARS M., M.D. **STOCKTON** • SAFFIER, SHERMAN F., M.D. • GRIFFITHS, HAROLD M., M.D. **SUNLAND** • SAMARRAI, LABIB A. R., M.D. **TARZANA** • STEIN, KARL N., M.D. **THOUSAND OAKS** • HENJYOJI, EDWARD Y., M.D. • PARDUE, A. MICHAEL, M.D. **TORRANCE** • McKISSOCK, PAUL K., M.D. • ROSENFIELD, HAROLD A., M.D. • STEEN, ALAN M., M.D. • SUTTERFIELD, THOMAS C., M.D. • THORRENS, SHELDON J., M.D. **TRUCKEE/NORTH LAKE TAHOE** • HOLDERNESS, HOWARD, JR., M.D. **TUSTIN** • RAPPAPORT, I., M.D. **VACAVILLE** • JONES, FREDERICK R., M.D. **VAN NUYS** • BARKER, DONALD E., M.D. **VENTURA** • ARMSTRONG, DALE P., M.D. **WALNUT CREEK** • BOROCZ, ISTVAN, M.D. • DELGADO, CARLOS G., M.D. • GRAY, GERALD N., M.D. • JERVIS, WILLIAM, M.D. **WEST COVINA** • MURPHY, JOHN E., M.D. • SANCHEZ, SERGIO M., M.D. **WESTLAKE VILLAGE** • SENGELMANN, ROBERT P., M.D. • SLYWKA, BRIAN H., M.D. • TERINO, EDWARD O., M.D. **WOODLAND HILLS** • FISHER, WILLIAM J., M.D. **WOODSIDE** • WEBER, JAROY, JR., M.D.

COLORADO

AURORA • EISENBAUM, SIDNEY L., M.D. • GROSSMAN, JOHN A., M.D. • POWERS, WILLIAM E., JR., M.D. **BOULDER** • KLOSTER, GILBERT J., M.D. • STORMO, ALAN C., M.D. **COLORADO SPRINGS** • BANCROFT, GEORGE W., M.D. • DuBOIS, DAVID D., M.D. • HANSON, JEROME R., M.D. • SPEIRS, ALFRED C., M.D. **DENVER** • BETSON, RAYMOND J., JR., M.D. • BLANFORD, SIDNEY E., M.D. • FAWELL, THOMAS W., M.D. • GARCIA, F. A., M.D. • GILL, JOHN R., M.D. • HECKLER, FREDERICK R., M.D. • HOEHN, ROBERT J., M.D. • LILLA, JAMES A., M.D. • MACOMBER, DOUGLAS W., M.D. • McKINNON, DOUGLAS A., M.D. • RICH, JOHN D., M.D. • RODRIGUEZ, JOSE L., M.D. • VIGOR,

151

WILLIAM N., M.D. • WEATHERLY-WHITE, R. C. A., M.D. • ZBYLSKI, JOSEPH R., M.D. **ENGLEWOOD** • LACY, GEORGE M., M.D. **FORT COLLINS** • SMITH, KIRK M., M.D. **GRAND JUNCTION** • MERKEL, WILLIAM D., M.D. **LAKEWOOD** • VIGOR, WILLIAM N., M.D. **LITTLETON** • KNIZE, DAVID M., M.D. **PUEBLO** • LAWRENCE, RICHARD A., M.D. • SIEMSEN, GERALD H., M.D. **WESTMINSTER** • TEGTMEIER, RONALD E., M.D. **WHEAT RIDGE** • MARA, JOHN E., M.D.

CONNECTICUT

BRIDGEPORT • CALABRESE, CARMINE T., M.D. • CORSO, PHILIP F., M.D. **DANBURY** • FISCHL, ROBERT A., M.D. **GREENWICH** • FODOR, PETER B., M.D. **HARTFORD** • BAB-COCK, ALBERT L., M.D. • BASS, DAVID M., M.D. • BROWN, STEPHEN A., M.D. • JONES, WILLIAM D., III, M.D. • KELLY, CLAUDE C., M.D. • PLATT, JOAN M., M.D. • SMITH, LEONARD K., M.D. **MERIDEN** • FRANCESCON, SERGIO D., M.D. **NEW HAVEN** • ARIYAN, STEPHAN, M.D. • ARONS, MARVIN S., M.D. • CLIMO, SAMUEL, M.D. • FINSETH, FREDERICK J., M.D. • FLAGG, STEPHEN V., M.D. • FRAZIER, WILLIAM H., M.D. • KOSS, NEAL, M.D. • KRIZEK, THOMAS J., M.D. • MOMBELLO, GARY E., M.D. • POLAYES, IRVING M., M.D. **NEW LONDON** • HOSTNIK, WILLIAM J., M.D. **NORWALK** • SINGER, JOEL B., M.D. **OLD GREENWICH** • REIN, JOEL M., M.D. **STAMFORD** • GEER, E. THROOP, M.D. **WATERBURY** • KOSTECKI, RICHARD J., M.D. • WOHLGEMUTH, PAUL R., M.D.

DELAWARE

NEWARK • HOCHBERG, JULIO, M.D. **WILMINGTON** • DeLEEUW, NEIL A., M.D. • GRAY, H. WENDELL, JR., M.D. • KIM, KYO A., M.D. • METZGER, JAMES T., M.D. • SAUNDERS, DAVID E., M.D.

DISTRICT OF COLUMBIA

WASHINGTON • DICK, ARTHUR, M.D. • FLEURY, ALBERT F., M.D. • KEUNEN, HUGO F., M.D. • LeFLORE, IVENS C., M.D. • LETTERMAN, GORDON S., M.D. • LITTON, CLYDE, M.D. • MAGASSY, CSABA L., M.D. • PARSONS, ROBERT W., M.D. • SCHURTER, MAXINE ANN, M.D. • THOMPSON, LEWIS W., M.D. • WILENSKY, ROBERT J., M.D. • WILSON, ROBERT M., M.D. • ZAMICK, PAUL, M.D.

FLORIDA

ALTAMONTE SPRINGS • BECK, RICHARD L., M.D. • NAZARETH, RICHARD M., M.D. **BOCA RATON** • PERSOFF, MYRON M., M.D. **BRADENTON** • CAMPBELL, ROSS, M.D. **CLEARWATER** • BROWN, KENNETH P., III, M.D. • WELLS, ROBERT L., JR., M.D. **CORAL GABLES** • MILLER, ROBERT F., M.D. • NORMAN, HAROLD G., M.D. • SWENSEN, FREDERICK C., M.D. **DAVIE** • JOSEPH, JULIUS M., M.D. **DAYTONA BEACH** • HERRERO, FRANCISCO A., M.D. **FORT LAUDERDALE** • BIRNBAUM, JON JAY, M.D. • BOLT, DONALD A., M.D. • BONURA, CHARLES M., M.D. • HOGAN, WILLIAM F., M.D. • SEROPIAN, DIRAN, M.D. • SMITH, ROBERT B., M.D. **FORT MYERS** • BRUNO, JOHN S., M.D. • DOWD, JAMES F., M.D. **GAINESVILLE** • BINGHAM, HAL G., M.D. • FURLOW, LEONARD T., JR., M.D. • HABAL, MUTAZ B., M.D. • HOGUE, ROBERT J., JR., M.D. • WALTON, BRUCE E., M.D. **HIGHLAND BEACH** • HUGHES, WENDELL L., M.D. **HOLLANDALE** • SHERMAN, STANLEY, M.D. **HOLLYWOOD** • FABRIC, ROBERT K., M.D. • SHUSTER, MARVIN M., M.D. • WALD, HARLAN I., M.D. **JACKSONVILLE** • DUNCAN, ROBERT E., M.D. • DUSHOFF, IRA M., M.D. • FINK, GEORGE H., M.D. • KAYE, BERNARD L., M.D. • MORGAN, BERNARD L., M.D. • OBI, LEWIS J., M.D. • ROSENTHAL, SAMUEL G., M.D. • SNOW, JOHN W., M.D. **LAKE WORTH** • REDDY, KRIS M., M.D. **MELBOURNE** • REMARK, FREDERICK L., M.D. **MIAMI** • BAKER, THOMAS J., M.D. • BASS, CRAIG B., M.D. • DEVINE, JOHN W., JR., M.D. • GARST, WALTER P., M.D. • GEORGE, PHILLIP T., M.D. • GORDON, HOWARD L., M.D. • LEVINE, GEORGE A., M.D. • LITTLE, JOHN W., III, M.D. • MEM-BERY, JOAN H., M.D. • MILLARD, D. RALPH, JR., M.D. • MONAL, MANUEL A., M.D. • MULLIN, WALTER R., M.D. • NORMAN, JACK D., M.D. • RAPPERPORT, ALAN S., M.D. • ROBERTSON, GEORGE W., M.D. • ROBERTSON, JAMES G., M.D. • SNYDER, GILBERT B., M.D. • STOKLEY, SAMUEL P. H., M.D. • TALARICO, DAVID J., M.D. • THOMPSON, IAN D., M.D. • WOLFE, S. ANTHONY, M.D. • ZAHLER, CHARLES G., M.D. • ZAYDON, THOMAS J., M.D. • ZUFI, DAVID, M.D. **MIAMI BEACH** • ROBBINS, LAWRENCE B., M.D. • SAFIAN, JOSEPH, M.D. **MIAMI SHORES** • KITSOS, CONSTANTINE N., M.D. **NAPLES** • MOGELVANG, L. CHRISTIAN, M.D. **NORTH MIAMI BEACH** • ELLENBY, JAY D., M.D. • FREIMAN, MORTON E., M.D. • RADLAUER, CHARLES B., M.D. • RODRIQUEZ, J. REMON, M.D. • TRUPPMAN, EDWARD S., M.D. **ORLANDO** • BAKER, JAMES L., JR., M.D. • BARTELS, ROGER J., M.D. • DOUGLAS, WILLIAM M., M.D. **PALM BEACH GARDENS** • WHALEN, WILLIAM P., M.D. **PENSACOLA** • GREGORY, BEN T., M.D. • ORTEGA, TEODORO K., M.D. • SCHLICHTER, FRANK J., JR., M.D. **PLANTATION** • ZELMAN, DONALD, M.D. **POMPANO BEACH** • MAYL, NATHAN, M.D. **ST. PETERSBURG** • AUSTIN, GROVER W., M.D. • HAMILTON, JOHN M., M.D. • MEJIA-MILLAN, SILVIO, M.D. • PHARES, RICHARD E., M.D. **SARASOTA** • BRYANT, W. MICHAEL, M.D. • HILL, CHARLES H., M.D. • WILSON, LEO H., JR., M.D. **SOUTH MIAMI** • BALCH, CLYDE R., M.D. • LEVIN, JOEL M., M.D. **STUART** • BASS, HAROLD M., M.D. • RANDALL, ROBERT G., M.D. **TALLAHASSEE** • McKINNEY, MEREDITH, M.D. • MOORE, CHARLES E., M.D. **TAMPA** • DUBIN, DALE B., M.D. • LIU, VICTOR K. Y., M.D. • MATTISON, JOEL W. L., M.D. • NOVICK, MAURICE, M.D. • TAYLOR, WILLIAM G., M.D. **WEST PALM BEACH** • ALFONSO, ALVARO, M.D. • CRAFT, JEROME W., M.D. • ELMQUIST, JOHN G., M.D. • WEYBRIGHT, DORTHEA, M.D. **WINTER PARK** • OHLWILER, DAVID A., M.D. • ROYER, JOHN P., M.D.

GEORGIA

ATLANTA • BLACK, PAUL W., M.D. • BOSTWICK, JOHN III, M.D. • BROWN, ROBERT G., M.D. • CROW, ROBERT W., M.D. • GRIFFIN, JOHN M., M.D. • HAMM, WILLIAM G.,

M.D. • HARTLEY, JOHN H., JR., M.D. • HARTRAMPF, CARL R., M.D. • HOBBY, LOVIC W., M.D. • HUGER, WILLIAM E., JR., M.D. • JURKIEWICZ, MAURICE J., M.D. • LEWIS, JOHN R., M.D. • MATTISON, RICHARD C., M.D. • MUNNA, JOHN C., M.D. • POUND, EDWIN C., JR., M.D. • RUSSELL, R. JAMES, M.D. • SCHATTEN, WILLIAM E., M.D. • SLUTSKY, MORTON, M.D. • VASCONEZ, LUIS O., M.D. • WEISS, HARVEY A., M.D. • YARN, CHARLES P., JR., M.D. **AUGUSTA** • FLANAGIN, W. S., M.D. • STILL, JOSEPH M., JR., M.D. **AUSTELL** • FEINERMAN, MICHAEL B., M.D. **BRUNSWICK** • DIXON, JIMMY L., M.D. **COLUMBUS** • VAN DUYN, JOHN, M D. **DECATUR** • CARSPECKEN, H. HUTSON, M.D. • LEONARD, ROBERT P., M.D. • WHITSON, THEODORE C., M.D. **EAST POINT** • RUSCA, JOHN A., M.D. **FORT GORDON** • BECKWITH, MERTON M., M.D. **GROVETOWN** • MAYER, D. McCULLAGH, M.D. **MACON** • FREEMAN, RONALD A., M.D. • MAGNAN, CHARLES G., JR., M.D. **MARIETTA** • MUSARRA, ELMER A., II, M.D. • WOFFORD, BENJAMIN H., JR., M.D. **SAVANNAH** • FINGER, E. RONALD, M.D.

HAWAII

AIEA • LAU, BENNETT M. K., M.D. **HONOLULU** • FERNANDEZ, LEABERT R., M.D. • FLOWERS, ROBERT S., M.D. • HAY-ROE, VICTOR, M.D. • JIM, VERNON K., M.D. • KUBO, KATSUJI, M.D. • McDOWELL, FRANK, M.D. • PENOFF, JAMES, M.D. • SIEGEL, RICHARD J., M.D. • TAIRA, TOM K., M.D.

IDAHO

BOISE • HAYES, J. EDWARD, M.D. • SULLIVAN, C. EUGENE, M.D.

ILLINOIS

M.D. • ROSENBERG, DALE H., M.D. • SALYAPONGSE, AMORN, M.D. • TSCHOE, BJONG-**ARLINGTON HEIGHTS** • KNODE, ROBERT E., M.D. **BELLEVILLE** • MAUN, LORENZO P., SUHN, M.D. **CHICAGO** • ASHBELL, T. SHELLY, M.D. • BEERS, MORRISON D., M.D. • BERGER, JACK C., M.D. • BRADLEY, CRAIG, M.D. • BROWN, J. VICKERS, M.D. • CURTIN, JOHN WILLIAM, M.D. • EDSTROM, LEE E., M.D. • FEINBERG, LILLA A., M.D. • FISHER, DAVID, M.D. • GREELEY, PAUL W., M.D. • GRIFFITH, B. HEROLD, M.D. • HASRAJANI, MANOHAR U., M.D. • HUGO, NORMAN E., M.D. • JAYARAM, BANGALORE N., M.D. • KAVKA, STEPHEN J., M.D. • KURTH, MILTON E., M.D. • LANDA, STUART J. F., M.D. • LEWIS, NOLAN S., M.D. • LOPEZ, ENRIQUE M., M.D. • LUANGKESORN, PRASERT, M.D. • McKINNEY, PETER W., M.D. • McNALLY, RANDALL E., M.D. • PICK, JOHN F., M.D. • ROBSON, MARTIN C., M.D. • ROSS, DAVID A., M.D. • SCHENCK, ROBERT R., M.D. • SLAUGHTER, WAYNE B., M.D. • SPRINGER, HARRY A., M.D. • STONE, NELSON H., M.D. • SWARTZ, ROBERT M., M.D. • TANSKI, EUGENE V., M.D. • TASCHE, CONRAD, M.D. **ELGIN** • SHEDBALKAR, A. R., M.D., **EVANSTON** • PIRRUCCELLO, FRANK W., M.D. • RANDOLPH, DAVID A., M.D. • SULLIVAN, MARTIN R., M.D. **GLENVIEW** • ROSEN-BERG, JAY H., M.D. **GURNEE** • ATZEFF, LUBEN, M.D. **HINSDALE** • SOHAEY, MANUTCHEHR, M.D. **JOLIET** • TSAI, VINCENTE T. NG., M.D. **LA GRANGE** • NAWADA, CHANNAKESHAVA U., M.D. • STOKES, ROBERT F., M.D. **LAKE FOREST** • STEINWALD, OSMAR P., JR., M.D. **LIBERTYVILLE** • BAER, HENRY A., M.D. **MAYWOOD** • MONAS-TERIO, JACK M., M.D. • WARPEHA, RAYMOND L., M.D. **MOLINE** • FERDINANDS, MICHAEL C., M.D. **MT. PROSPECT** • McLean, ALLEN D., M.D. **NAPIERVILLE** • LEARY, EDWARD J., M.D. **OAKBROOK** • BADRI, A. ALLEN, M.D. • JANDA, CHARLES A., M.D. **OAK FOREST** • ARUMUGAM, SUBRAMANIAM, M.D. • JAYASANKER, M. R., M.D. **OAK LAWN** • SEETAPUN, ANUN, M.D. **OAK PARK** • ANGELATS, JUAN, M.D. **PARK RIDGE** • SCHULTZ, RICHARD C., M.D. • SEATON, J. RALPH, JR., M.D. **PEORIA** • CORLEY, RICHARD D., M.D. • RICHARDSON, ROBERT J., M.D. **RIVER FOREST** • FELIX, ERNEST R., M.D. **ROCKFORD** • BADER, KARL F., JR., M.D. • JOHNSON, HUGH A., M.D. • WEIS-KOPF, JEROME S., M.D. **ST. CHARLES** • McKENZIE, MARY L., M.D. **SCOTT AIR FORCE BASE** • BERNSTEN, STEPHEN, M.D. **SKOKIE** • SPERLING, RICHARD L., M.D. **SPRING-FIELD** • WAVAK, PAUL W., M.D. • ZOOK, ELVIN G., M.D. **WAUKEGAN** • RYAN, ROBERT A., M.D. **WOODRIDGE** • QUINTERO, EDGAR A., M.D.

INDIANA

EVANSVILLE • PULCINI, JOHN D., M.D. **FORT WAYNE** • BRUCKER, PERRY A., M.D. • FURTADO, ROBERT, M.D. • HULL, DeWAYNE L., M.D. **INDIANAPOLIS** • BAUER, THOMAS B., M.D. • BENNETT, JAMES, M.D. • HUGHES, CHARLES E., III, M.D. • MAYER, JOHN RONALD, M.D. • MONN, LARRY N., M.D. • MOORE, THOMAS S., M.D. • PANTZER, JOHN G., JR., M.D. • QAZI, HAROON M., M.D. • RABER, ROBERT M., M.D. • SENTANY, MARKI S., M.D. • TONDRA, JOHN M., M.D. • TRUSLER, H. MARSHALL, M.D. **MERRILL-VILLE** • ZUCKER, EDWARD, M.D. **MUNSTER** • GOLDENBERG, MITCHELL E., M.D. **SOUTH BEND** • BOOTH, FRANKLIN MILLER, M.D. • MAUZY, MERRITT C., M.D.

IOWA

DES MOINES • STALLINGS, JAMES O., III, M.D. • WOODBURN, BOYNTON T., M.D. **IOWA CITY** • McSHANE, RICHARD H., M.D. **WATERLOO** • AHRENHOLZ, DONALD J., M.D.

KANSAS

KANSAS CITY • HARDIN, CREIGHTON A., M.D. • KETCHUM, LYNN D., M.D. • MASTERS, FRANCIS W., M.D. • ROBINSON, DAVID W., M.D. **PRAIRIE VILLAGE** • NOSTI, JUAN C., M.D. • YE, RICHARD C., M.D. • YOUNG, JOHN W., M.D. **SHAWNEE MISSION** • SAFFO, K. S., M.D. **TOPEKA** • BETHEA, HARDEE, M.D. • HUTTON, FREDERICK A., M.D. • KELLEY, JAMES W., M.D. **WICHITA** • FERRIS, BRUCE G., M.D. • HIEBERT, A. E., M.D. • KENDALL, TOM EDWARD, M.D. • NELSON, GERALD D., M.D. • PULLMAN, HORMAN KEITH, M.D. • REMPEL, JOHN H., M.D. • SHAW, RICHARD C., M.D.

KENTUCKY

LEXINGTON • ARCHER, RALEIGH R., M.D. • COATS, THOMAS F., M.D. • LUCE, EDWARD A., M.D. • MOORE, ANDREW M., M.D. • MULDROW, LOUIS M., JR., M.D. **LOUISVILLE** • COLE, NORMAN M., M.D. • GIANNINI, J. THOMAS, M.D. • HAGAN, THOMAS W., M.D. • KASDAN, MORTON L., M.D. • KINCAID, CHARLES A., M.D. • LENEHAN, JOSEPH M., M.D. • LISTER, GRAHAM D., M.D. • STAMBAUGH, HARRY D., M.D. • VERDI, GERALD D., M.D. • WEETER, JOHN C., M.D. • WEINER, LEONARD J., M.D. • WOLFE, JOHN J., M.D. **MADISONVILLE** • WAYNE, LISLE, II, M.D.

LOUISIANA

BATON ROUGE • BELL, MARTIN L., M.D. • ENGERON, O'NEIL, M.D. • KISNER, WENDELL H., M.D. • MOORE, KAY, M.D. **LAFAYETTE** • CROMWELL, TERRY A., M.D. • HENDERSON, DARRELL L., M.D. **METAIRIE** • OWENS, A. NEAL, M.D. **MONROE** • WORTHEN, EUGENE F., M.D. **NEW ORLEANS** • CHURCH, JOHN M., JR., M.D. • COLON, GUSTAVO A., M.D. • DELGADO, DELIO DAVID, M.D. • DIEFFENBACH, KENNETH M., M.D. • HOFFMAN, GEORGE W., M.D. • KRUST, LOUIS, M.D. • MASSIHA, HAMID, M.D. • McKEE, DUNCAN M., M.D. • MEADE, ROBERT J., M.D. • POLLOCK, WILLIAM J., M.D. • RYAN, ROBERT F., M.D. **SHREVEPORT** • BUTLER, LEWELL C., M.D. • GRAHAM, JOHN K., M.D. • VALIULIS, JOHN P., M.D. • WALL, SIMEON H., M.D.

MAINE

PORTLAND • LABELLE, JEAN J., M.D. • OLMSTED, BURTON L., M.D. **SOUTH PORTLAND** • MacDOUGAL, BRUCE A., M.D.

MARYLAND

BALTIMORE • BALLESTEROS, RUBEN F., M.D. • BERG, ELLIOTT M., M.D. • DAVIS, WM. BOWDOIN, M.D. • HANSEN, FREDERIK C., JR., M.D. • McGIBBON, BERNARD M., M.D. • PINKNER, LAWRENCE D., M.D. • PLASSE, JEROME S., M.D. • SU, CHI-TSUNG, M.D. • VAHOS, MARIO, M.D. **BETHESDA** • CAMERON, RONALD R., M.D. • COLGAN, DIANE L., M.D. • DEMPSEY, WILLIAM C., M.D. • DOWLING, JOHN A., M.D. • HAVERBACK, CHESTER Z., M.D. • LATHAM, WILBUR D., M.D. • METZ, PHILIP S., M.D. **GAITHERSBURG** • CONRAD, ROBERT N., M.D. **GLEN BURNIE** • MEHLER, GEORGE J., M.D. **HAGERSTOWN** • CLARK, JOHN WILSON, M.D. • HAYNES, AUBREY F., M.D. • TUMBUSCH, WILFRED T., M.D. **HUNT VALLEY** • HOOPES, JOHN E., M.D. • RYAN, JAMES J., M.D. **LUTHERVILLE** • JASION, ARTHUR R., M.D. **PIKESVILLE** • KLATSKY, STANLEY A., M.D. **ROCKVILLE** • TEIMOURIAN, BEHMAN, M.D. **SALISBURY** • LARGE, OCTAVUS P., M.D. **SEVERNA PARK** • CONVERSE, CHARLES F., M.D. **SILVER SPRING** • AZZATO, NICHOLAS M., M.D. • ENG, JOHN S., M.D. • KOURY, THOMAS L., M.D. • RATINO, JOHN M., M.D. • REISIN, JORGE H., M.D. • SHANOFF, LESLIE B., M.D. **TOWSON** • ORLANDO, JOSEPH C., M.D. • WILHELMSEN, HANS R., M.D.

MASSACHUSETTS

BEVERLY • PATEL, MAHESH M., M.D. **BOSTON** • ANASTASI, GASPAR W., M.D. • CANNON, BRADFORD, M.D. • COCHRAN, THOMAS C., M.D. • CONSTABLE, JOHN D., M.D. • GIFFORD, GEORGE H., JR., M.D. • GOLDWYN, ROBERT M., M.D. • LEWIS, MICHAEL B., M.D. • MacCOLLUM, DONALD W., M.D. • MARSHALL, KENNETH A., M.D. • MAY, JAMES W., JR., M.D. • MULLIKEN, JOHN B., M.D. • MURRAY, JOSEPH E., M.D. • NOE, JOEL M., M.D. • PARRY, RICHARD G., M.D. • REMENSNYDER, JOHN P., M.D. • SOHN, STEPHEN A., M.D. • WOLFORT, FRANCIS G., M.D. • WYSOCKI, JOHN P., M.D. **BREWSTER** • DALAND ERNEST M., M.D. **CAMBRIDGE** • FELDMAN, JOEL J., M.D. **CONCORD** • PANTAZELOS, HYTHO H., M.D. • WINSTEN, JOSEPH, M.D. **FRAMINGHAM** • DELMAN, ALAN, M.D. **LYNN** • MITCHELL, ELMER T., JR., M.D. • VALLIS, CHARLES P., M.D. **MEDFORD** • FRIEDMAN, STEVEN J., M.D. **MILTON** • O'BRIEN, ROBERT W., M.D. **NEW BEDFORD** • KELLEHER, ROBERT E., M.D. • McCARTHY, LAWRENCE J., M.D. **NEWTON LOWER FALLS** • COURTISS, EUGENE H., M.D. • DAVIDSON, BARRY A., M.D. • WEBSTER, RICHARD C., M.D. **NORTH ANDOVER** • SCULLY, STEPHEN J., M.D. **NORTH DARTMOUTH** • RUGGIERO, NOVELLO E., M.D. **NORWOOD** • BECKER, MARTIN D., M.D. • O'BRIEN, JOHN J., M.D. **PEABODY** • MOORE, WILLIAM R., M.D. **PITTSFIELD** • STERN, ORRIN, S., M.D. **SPRINGFIELD** • BAKER, JOSEPH M., M.D. • MILLER, RICHARD J., M.D. • STODDARD, PHILIP B., M.D. • STONE, PHILIP A., M.D. • TRAUB, ABRAHAM, M.D. **WELLESLEY** • O'SULLIVAN, RENEE BENNETT, M.D. **WINCHESTER** • VIRNELLI, FRANK R., M.D. **WORCESTER** • BACCHETTA, CARLOS A., M.D. • BOM, ADRIAN F., M.D. • CHANG, WALLACE H. J., M.D. • CONNORS, DAVID W., M.D.

MICHIGAN

ANN ARBOR • BUCKO, C. DENNIS, M.D. • DINGMAN, REED O., M.D. • GRABB, WILLIAM C., M.D. • MARKLEY, JOHN M., JR., M.D. • ONEAL, ROBERT M., M.D. **BIRMINGHAM** • CARLISLE, JOSEPH D., M.D. • POOL, ROBERT, M.D. • JACOBSON, HERBERT S., M.D. **DETROIT** • DITMARS, DONALD M., JR., M.D. • HILL, EDWARD J., JR., M.D. • KELLY, ALEX P., JR., M.D. • LANGE, WILLIAM A., M.D. • McEVITT, WILLIAM G., M.D. • STEFANI, ANDREW E., M.D. • WEISSMAN, FREDRICK, M.D. • WINKELMAN, NED Z., M.D. **EAST LANSING** • CONSTANT, ERRIKOS, M.D. • DAVIS, DON G., M.D. • GOMEZ, JORGE, M.D. **FLINT** • PIPER, W. ARCHIBALD, M.D. • POOMEE, AMORN, M.D. • TARRANT, LAWRENCE W., M.D. **GRAND RAPIDS** • BEERNINK, JOHN, M.D. • BIRKBECK, BENJAMIN H., M.D. • BLOCKSMA, RALPH, M.D. • SEBRIGHT, JOHN A., M.D. • SIMPSON, WILLIAM D., M.D. • STEFFENSEN, W. H., M.D. • YOST, WILLIAM G., JR., M.D. **GROSSE POINTE WOODS** • McCABE, W. PETER, M.D. **KALAMAZOO** • DORNER, KENNETH R., M.D. • NEWMAN, FRANK J., M.D. • RAMOS, HERNANDO, M.D. **MUSKEGON** • GRENNAN,

LAWRENCE E., M.D. **NORTH MUSKEGON** • KISLOV, RICHARD, M.D. **ROYAL OAK** • CARLISLE, JOSEPH D., M.D. • GELLIS, MICHAEL B., M.D. • ORDONA, ROBINSON U., M.D. • RAM, SRI R., M.D. **SAGINAW** • CRESSWELL, THOMAS A., M.D. • VALIA, SAMUEL S., M.D. **SOUTHFIELD** • HAWTOF, DAVID B., M.D. • HIPPS, C. J., M.D. • KAPETANSKY, DONALD I., M.D. • LAWSON, JAMES M., M.D. • NEWBY, BURNS G., M.D. • STRAITH, RICHARD E., M.D. **TROY** • JAFFE, HAROLD W., M.D. • WALLACE, DONALD B., M.D.

MINNESOTA

MINNEAPOLIS • CHESLER, MERRILL D., M.D. • DODD, ROSALIE M., M.D. • GAVISER, JAMES B., M.D. • KRAGH, LYLE V., M.D. • LUKINAC, CHARLES J., M.D. • SHONS, ALAN R., M.D. • STEVENS, SHERIDAN S. H., M.D. • VOGT, PETER A., M.D. **ROCHESTER** • ARNOLD, PHILIP G., M.D. • DEVINE, KENNETH D., M.D. • ERICH, JOHN B., M.D. • IRONS, GEORGE B., JR., M.D. • LITZOW, T. J., M.D. • MASSON, JAMES K., M.D. • WOODS, JOHN E., M.D. **ST. PAUL** • MacDONALD, CHARLES J., M.D. • MESSENGER, MICHAEL A., M.D. • PILNEY, FRANK T., M.D. • STAFNE, JOHN G., M.D.

MISSISSIPPI

BILOXI • EDWARDS, JOHN B., M.D. **GREENVILLE** • LOVE, ROBERT T., JR., M.D. **JACK-SON** • BOBO, WILLIAM O., M.D. • ETHRIDGE, HEBER C., SR., M.D. • GODFREY, W. DOUGLAS, M.D. • JABALEY, MICHAEL, M.D. • SMITH, ROBERT A., M.D. • SONG-CHAROEN, SOMPRASONG, M.D.

MISSOURI

COLUMBIA • HEIMBURGER, RICHARD A., M.D. • KAPLAN, MICHAEL F., M.D. • PUCKETT, CHARLES L., M.D. • REDDY, R. RAMACHANDRA, M.D. **INDEPENDENCE** • MOSBACHER, HUGH E., M.D. **KANSAS CITY** • ABEND, MELVIN N., M.D. • CHANDLER, ROBERT A., M.D. • COLEMAN, ROBERT L., M.D. • CROW, MARTIN L., M.D. • GASKINS, JOHN H., M.D. • GUTEK, E. PHILIP, M.D. • HOPKINS, JAMES P., M.D. • McCOY, FREDERICK J., M.D. • MORGAN, W. RICHARD, JR., M.D. • WEBB, HARRY E., M.D. **ST. LOUIS** • BANJASTITKUL, CHUSAK, M.D. • BROWN, RICHARD J. C., M.D. • CHAMNESS, JAMES T., M.D. • EADES, JOSEPH W., M.D. • FELICIANO, WILFRIDO C., M.D. • FRYER, MINOT P., M.D. • HALFORD, RICHARD M., M.D. • HOLTMANN, BARBEL, M.D. • JOHN-SON, CHARLES J., M.D. • LISCHER, CARL E., M.D. • LISSNER, ARTHUR BART, M.D. • ONKEN, HENRY DRALLE, M.D. • PALLETA, F. X., M.D. • PAPPALARDO, CARLOS, M.D. • PAYNE, MEREDITH JORSTAD, M.D. • RIBAUDO, J. MICHAEL, M.D. • STONEMAN, WILLIAM, III, M.D. • WEBBER, WILLIAM B., M.D. • WEEKS, PAUL M., M.D. • WHITE, BRUCE I., M.D. • WRAY, R. CHRISTIE, JR., M.D. • ZOGRAFAKIS, GEORGE H., M.D. **SPRINGFIELD** • DOMANN, DARREL D., M.D. • GASKA, WALTER J., M.D. • WINSKY, ARLEN D., M.D.

MONTANA

BILLINGS • GALLOWAY, DWIGHT V., M.D. • PEET, WALTER J., M.D. **BUTTE** • GUTSTEIN, ROBERT A., M.D. **GREAT FALLS** • NOVARK, BRUCE W., M.D. • O'CONNOR, JOHN E., M.D. **MISSOULA** • MURRAY, DONALD E., M.D.

NEBRASKA

LINCOLN • LeWORTHY, G. WILLIAM, M.D. • RUTH, LARRY D., M.D. **OMAHA** • BACCARI, M. EDWARD, M.D. • BLACK, ALBERT S., M.D. • DAHL, CARL H., M.D. • THOMPSON, CHESTER Q., JR., M.D.

NEVADA

CARSON CITY • CHAMPION, WILLIAM J., M.D. **LAS VEGAS** • BONGIOVI, JOSEPH J., JR., M.D. • DOMBROWSKI, DONALD J., M.D. • KOPF, EDWARD HENRY, M.D. • VINNIK, CHARLES A., M.D. **RENO** • GREENBERG, GEORGE H., M.D. • ILIESCU, JOHN, JR., M.D. • STRAND, GARETH W., M.D.

NEW HAMPSHIRE

HANOVER • BROWN, FORST E., M.D. • MORAIN, WILLIAM D., M.D. • RUECKERT, FREDERIC, M.D. • TANZER, RADFORD C., M.D. **MANCHESTER** • PACIK, PETER THOMAS, M.D.

NEW JERSEY

BLOOMINGDALE • KOSTECKI, JOSEPH L., M.D. **CHERRY HILL** • KRAUSE, JOHN L., JR., M.D. • LUDIN, EDWARD N., M.D. **CLIFTON** • PECK, GEORGE C., M.D. **COLLINGSWOOD** • VON DEILEN, ARTHUR W., M.D. **EAST ORANGE** • AMR, MAHMOUD A., M.D. • LO-VERME, STEPHEN R., M.D. **EDISON** • ARKOULAKIS, STAMATIS E., M.D. **ENGLEWOOD** • BAXT, SHERWOOD A., M.D. **FAIR LAWN** • BLOOMENSTEIN, RICHARD B., M.D. **JERSEY CITY** • REDDY, LOKA N., M.D. **LIVINGSTON** • BRIGGS, ROBERT M., M.D. • KEYSER, JOHN J., M.D. • MEIJER, ROBBY, M.D. • PEER, LYNDON A., M.D **MONTCLAIR** • CONROY, WILLIAM C., M.D. **MORRISTOWN** • BERSCHADSKY, MARIO, M.D. • MALTON, S. DONALD, M.D. **NEPTUNE CITY** • RYAN, WALTER M., JR., M.D. **NEW BRUNSWICK** • GOLDSTEIN, MORTON HILL, M.D. • ROTHFLEISCH, SHELDON, M.D. **NORTHFIELD** • MONIHAN, RICHARD M., M.D. **PARAMUS** • GRECO, DANTE, M.D. **PASSAIC** • DeBELL, PETER J., M.D. **PLAINFIELD** • GRISWOLD, MERTON L., JR., M.D. • SAWHNEY, OM P., M.D. • STEINBERG, URSULA W., M.D. **PRINCETON** • BERAKHA, GEORGE J., M.D. • PUCHNER, GERHARD, M.D. • SNYDERMAN, REUVEN K., M.D. **RIDGEWOOD** • BAGLI, VINCENT J., M.D. • BOWE, JOHN J., M.D. **RIVER EDGE** • KRAISSL, CORNELIUS J., M.D. **SEA GIRT** • JASAITIS, JOSEPH S., M.D. **SHORT HILLS** • COESTER, FREDERICK G., M.D. **SOMERVILLE** • MARION, RUSSELL B., M.D. **TEANECK** • DiPIRRO, EARL J., M.D.

155

TOMS RIVER • BONGSADADT, TONGTIP, M.D. **TRENTON** • BABAR, ABDUL H., M.D. • DAVNE, ALBERT, M.D. **WEST ENGLEWOOD** • GOSSEL, JOHN D., M.D. **WESTFIELD** • SILVER, LESTER, M.D. **WEST ORANGE** • Di SPALTRO, FRANKLIN L., M.D. • FEEHAN, HUBERT F., M.D. • MANCUSI-UNGARO, ALVIN P., M.D.

NEW MEXICO

ALBUQUERQUE • BOVARD, CHARLES M., M.D. • COLOCHO, GUILERMO L., M.D. • GOODING, RICHARD A., M.D. • HERHAHN, FRANK T., M.D. • ORGEL, MICHAEL G., M.D. **SANTE FE** • MILLER, ROGER H., M.D.

NEW YORK

ALBANY • COLMAN, GERALD B., M.D. • ELLIOTT, RAY A., JR., M.D. • GREMINGER, RICHARD F., M.D. • HOEHN, JAMES G., M.D. • HOFFMEISTER, F. STANLEY, M.D. • MACOMBER, W. BRANDON, M.D. • STAYMAN, J. WEBSTER, III, M.D. • WANG, MARK K. H., M.D. **BARDONIA** • STORCH, MICHAEL D., M.D. **BETHPAGE** • EISEMAN, GILBERT, M.D. • TAURAS, ARVYDAS P., M.D. **BINGHAMPTON** • PEJO, SAMUEL P., M.D. • SUGUITAN, RODOLFO H., M.D. **BRONX** • ARGAMASO, RAVELO V., M.D. • DANILLER, AVRON I., M.D. • LEWIN, MICHAEL L., M.D. • MITHALAL, HARILAL, M.D. • OLLSTEIN, RONALD N., M.D. • STRAUCH, BERISH, M.D. • WEINER, DANIEL L., M.D. **BROOKLYN** • CANICK, M. LEON, M.D. • CRAMER, MARJORIE, M.D. • HARRIS, ALVIN H., M.D. • KLEIN, DANIEL, M.D. • MARKS, FREDRIC, M.D. • MINKOWITZ, FRANCES R., M.D. • RASI, HOWARD B., M.D. • REARDON, JAMES J., M.D. • SCHILLER, CARL, M.D. • TEPLITSKY, DAVID, M.D. • ULLOA, JOSE M., M.D. **BUFFALO** • BERMAN, HERBERT L., M.D. • CONNELLY, JOSEPH R., M.D. • DeFELICE, CLEMENT A., M.D. • DeKLEINE, E. HOYT, M.D. • GIUNTA, JOSEPH L., M.D. • HORWITZ, HANLEY M., M.D. • QUINLIVAN, JOHN K., M.D. • SHATKIN, SAMUEL, M.D. **CRANBERRY LAKE** • SUTTON, LEON E., M.D. **EAST MEADOW** • RUBIN, LEONARD R., M.D. **ELMIRA** • MARSHALL, JAMES H., M.D. • SONSIRE, JAMES M., M.D. **FOREST HILLS** • SCHESSEL, ELI S., M.D. **GARDEN CITY** • PENNISI, ANTHONY M., M.D. **GLENS FALLS** • KERCHNER, CLOYD C., M.D. **HEMPSTEAD, L. I.** • DUTT, NIHAR R., M.D. **HUNTINGTON** • ROTH, SAMUEL J., M.D. **IRVINGTON** • KIM, EUNG LIM, M.D. **JAMAICA** • CHASKO, STEPHEN G., M.D. **MINEOLA** • BROMBERG, B. E., M.D. • HERBSTRITT, JOSEPH G., M.D. • HERMANN, WALDEMAR F., M.D. • LEE, CHIN WOONG, M.D. • SONG, IN CHUL, M.D. • WALDEN, RICHARD H., M.D. • WISE, ARTHUR J., M.D. **NEW HYDE PARK** • BAZAN, CARLOS C., M.D. **NEW ROCHELLE** • CAPECI, THEODORE J., M.D. **NEW YORK** • ALTCHEK, EDGAR D., M.D. • ASHKAR, MICHAEL G., M.D. • ASTON, SHERRELL J., M.D. • AUFRICHT, GUSTAVE, M.D. • BALLANTYNE, LOWYD W. R., JR., M.D. • BARLOW, CARL MORTON, M.D. • BARSKY, ARTHUR J., M.D. • BEASLEY, ROBERT W., M.D. • BELLIN, HOWARD T., M.D. • BERRY, EDGAR P., M.D. • CASSON, PHILLIP R., M.D. • CHAGLASSIAN, TOROS A., M.D. • CINELLI, PETER B., M.D. • COBURN, RICHARD J., M.D. • CONVERSE, JOHN M., M.D. • COOPER, HOWARD, M.D. • COSMAN, BARD, M.D. • CRAIG, GEORGE T., M.D. • CRIKELAIR, GEORGE F., M.D. • DELGADO, JOSE P., M.D. • DOLICH, BARRY H., M.D. • DOMANSKIS, EDWARD J., M.D. • DUNAIF, CHARLES B., M.D. • DUNN, FRED S., M.D. • FISCHMAN, JEFFREY R., M.D. • GOULIAN, DICRAN, JR., M.D. • GILLEN, FRANCIS J., M.D. • GUTHRIE, RANDOLPH H., JR., M.D. • GUY, CARY L., M.D. • HERMAN, STEVEN, M.D. • HOFFMAN, SAUL, M.D. • HOGAN, V. MICHAEL, M.D. • HOLMSTRAND, KAJ E. H., M.D. • IMBER, GERALD, M.D. • JANECKA, IVO P., M.D. • JU, DAVID M. C., M.D. • KAHN, SIDNEY, M.D. • KAPLAN, JOSHUA M., M.D. • KOVACHEV, DANICA, M.D. • LeWINN, LAURENCE R., M.D. • LITTLER, J. WILLIAM, M.D. • MACDONALD, JAMES A., M.D. • MARTIN, HAYES E., M.D. • McCARTHY, JOSEPH G., M.D. • NORRIS, JAMES E. C., M.D. • OFODILE, FERDINAND A., M.D. • PORTER, VINCENT, M.D. • REES, THOMAS D., M.D. • RHOADS, HARMON T., JR., M.D. • RHODES, G. ANTHONY, M.D. • ROGERS, BLAIR O., M.D. • ROSENBERG, VICTOR I., M.D. • SCHER, CHARLES Z., M.D. • SCHER, SAMUEL L., M.D. • SCHULMAN, NORMAN H., M.D. • SCHWAGER, ROBERT G., M.D. • SEELEY, ROBERT C., M.D. • SHIP, ARTHUR G., M.D. • SIMON, BERNARD E., M.D. • SMITH, JAMES W., M.D. • STARK, RICHARD B., M.D. • STRIKER, PAUL S., M.D. • SYMONDS, FRANCIS C., JR., M.D. • TAUB, STANLEY, M.D. • TULENKO, JOHN F., M.D. • WASHIO, HIROSHI, M.D. • WESSER, DAVID R., M.D. • WEISS, PAUL R., M.D. • WOOD-SMITH, DONALD, M.D. • ZIMANY, ALEXANDER, M.D. **PATCHHOUGUE, L. I.** • TUERK, MILTON, M.D. **PLAINVIEW** • PIHL, BO GUNNAR A., M.D. **PORT JEFFERSON** • GRAFF, ARTHUR L., M.D. **POUGHKEEPSIE** • LAPIDUS, STEVEN M., M.D. • MacDOWELL, FREDERICK, JR., M.D. • SCILEPPI, ROBERT I., M.D. **RICHMOND HILL** • PRONO, ZAHIDE T., M.D. **ROCHESTER** • AGBAN, GALAA M., M.D. • ALLPORT, EDGAR L., M.D. • CALDWELL, ELETHEA H., M.D. • GEORGE, WARREN E., M.D. • KEPES, JOSEPH DRAY, M.D. • McCORMACK, ROBERT M., M.D. • READING, GEORGE P., M.D. • TOMASELLI, JOSEPH F., M.D. • VON KESSEL, FRED, M.D. **ROCKWELL CENTER** • DHALIWAL, AVTAR S., M.D. • MORRIS, JOEL J., M.D. **SCHENECTADY** • ADAMS, ARTHUR W., M.D. **SYRACUSE** • FALCONE, ALFRED E., M.D. • LEHRMAN, ARTHUR, M.D. • STARK, DAVID B., M.D. • STRUTHERS, ALFRED M., M.D. • SURITIS, ZIGURDS L., M.D. **TONAWANDA** • CALAMEL, PETER M., M.D. **TROY** • HACKER, LOUIS C., M.D. **UTICA** • SHAHEEN, ALBERT H., M.D. • TOKSU, ESAT A., M.D. **WHITE PLAINS** • BERNARD, ROBERT W., M.D. • BONANNO, PHILIP C., M.D. • DeHAAN, CLAYTON R., M.D. • MONTROY, ROBERT E., M.D. • MORELLO, DANIEL C., M.D. • SOLEY, ROBERT L., M.D. **WOODBURY** • LEEB, DIANNE C., M.D. **YONKERS** • MORRISSEY, MICHAEL F., M.D. • PELZER, RUDOLPH H., M.D.

NORTH CAROLINA

ASHEVILLE • ISRAEL, J. ROBERT, M.D. • LONGENECKER, CHARLES G., M.D. • McDOWELL, JAMES M., M.D. **CHAPEL HILL** • BEVIN, A. GRISWOLD, M.D. • TRIER,

WILLIAM C., M.D. **CHARLOTTE** • ALTANY, FRANKLIN E., M.D. • CHAPLIN, C. HAL, M.D. • GIBLIN, THOMAS R., M.D. • LAIRD, WILLIAM K., M.D. • MULLIS, WILLIAM F., M.D. • WALKER, ANDREW WILLIAM, M.D. **DURHAM** • GEORGIADE, NICHOLAS G., M.D. • PETERS, CALVIN R., M.D. • PICKRELL, KENNETH L., M.D. • SERAFIN, DONALD, M.D. • THOMPSON, LAWRENCE K., III, M.D. **FAYETTEVILLE** • FABIAN, DENIS, M.D. **GREENSBORO** • TANDON, MAHENDRA N., M.D. **GREENVILLE** • WALLACE, KELLEY, JR., M.D. **PINEHURST** • NEWTON, WALTER M., JR., M.D. **RALEIGH** • DAVIDIAN, VARTAN A., JR., M.D. • ROYSTER, HENRY P., M.D. • WINSLOW, ROBERT B., M.D. **WILMINGTON** • KROHN, JOHN R., M.D. **WINSTON-SALEM** • BEASON, EDWARD S., M.D. • GWYN, PAUL P., M.D. • HOWELL, JULIUS A., M.D.

NORTH DAKOTA

FARGO • LAMB, DONALD L., M.D.

OHIO

AKRON • CERVINO, A. LAWRENCE, M.D. • LEHMAN, JAMES A., JR., M.D. • LEWIS, JAMES M., M.D. • PRASAD, MANGALORE D., M.D. • SADDAWI, N. DAVID, M.D. • SANDEL, ALLAN J., M.D. **BEACHWOOD** • ARTZ, J. SHELDON, M.D. **CANTON** • KICOS, JOHN E., M.D. **CINCINNATI** • BOYER, BYRON E., M.D. • BROGAN, JOHN W., M.D. • CULLEN, DONAL S., M.D. • HANDLER, MARK B., M.D. • HYLAND, WILLIAM T., M.D. • KADIVAR, BAHRAM, M.D. • KAHL, JAMES B., M.D. • MARTIN, MARY M., M.D. • NEALE, HENRY W., M.D. • SLAGLE, ROBERT G., M.D. **CLEVELAND** • ANDERSON, ROBIN, M.D. • DES PREZ, JOHN D., M.D. • EARLE, A. SCOTT, M.D. • FLEEGLER, EARL J., M.D. • GLOVER, DONALD M., M.D. • HARTWELL, SHATTUCK W., JR., M.D. • JAFFE, STANLEY, M.D. • KIEHN, CLIFFORD L., M.D. • KURTAY, MINE A., M.D. • MANDEL, MARK A., M.D. • RICHEY, deWAYNE G., M.D. • SHAW, DARREL T., M.D. • SHAW, THOMAS E., M.D. **COLUMBUS** • BERGGREN, RONALD B., M.D. • BING, ARTHUR G. H., M.D. • DRABYN, GERALD A., M.D. • DURAN, ROBERT J., M.D. • FERRARO, JAMES W., II, M.D. • HOUSER, ROBERT G., M.D. • LEHV, MICHAEL S., M.D. • MAXWELL, CLARENCE L., M.D. • MOHLER, LESTER R., M.D. • NAILLE, RONALD A., M.D. • PORTERFIELD, H. WILLIAM, M.D. • POSTLEWAITE, DAVID S., M.D. • RUBERG, ROBERT L., M.D. • TERRY, JOHN L., M.D. • TRABUE, JOHN C., M.D. **DAYTON** • GRAUL, THOMAS C., M.D. • RAMNATH, RAMCHANDRA, M.D. • SNIDER, RALPH E., M.D. • WEISMAN, PHILIP A., M.D. • WELSH, GEORGE F., M.D. **GUYAHOGA FALLS** • AHMAD, MIRZA N., M.D. **LAKEWOOD** • SCARCELLA, JAMES V., M.D. **LORAIN** • FUSILERO, VICTORINO M., M.D. • MARFORI, NORBERTO R., M.D. **MAYFIELD HEIGHTS** • COAKWELL, CHARLES A., III, M.D. **MIDDLETOWN** • MUNICK, LEO H., M.D. **PARMA** • LI, CHARLES S., M.D. • RAUS, ELMER E., M.D. **RAVENNA** • KURI, ALIF A., M.D. **TOLEDO** • BAIBAK, GEORGE J., M.D. • DEAN, ROBERT K., M.D. • DILLER, JAMES G., M.D. • KELLEHER, JOHN C., M.D. • McWHORTER, HENRY E., M.D. • ROBINSON, JOHN H., M.D. • SADD, JOHN R., M.D. • SULLIVAN, JAMES G., M.D. **WAVERLY** • MONROE, CLARENCE W., M.D. **WILLOUGHBY** • BUKOVNIK, JOHN A., M.D. • TADDEO, RONALD J., M.D. **YOUNGSTOWN** • CHIU, YAU TOO, JR., M.D. • CUDDAPAH, SUBBARAYUDU, M.D. • DIETZ, GEORGE H., M.D. • MURRAY, RICHARD D., M.D.

OKLAHOMA

OKLAHOMA CITY • ANDERSON, HUBERT M., M.D. • BAJAJ, P. S., M.D. • BURTON, JOHN F., M.D. • DALTON, WILLIAM EDWARD, M.D. • FOERESTER, DAVID W., M.D. • FORREST, WILLIAM J., M.D. • HYROOP, GILBERT L., M.D. • KELLY, J. MICHAEL, M.D. • KIMBALL, GEORGE H., M.D. • KRAVITZ, HERBERT M., M.D. • McLAUGHLIN, ROBERT A., M.D. • SHADID, EDWARD A., M.D. • SILVERSTEIN, PAUL, M.D. **TULSA** • BROWN, LEONARD H., M.D. • CLARK, JOHN M., M.D. • FORREST, HERBERT J., M.D. • MARTIN, FRED R., M.D.

OREGON

BEND • NYE, JERRY E., M.D. **EUGENE** • CUTLER, RALPH GARR, M.D. • JARRETT, JOHN R., M.D. • TEAL, DONALD F., M.D. **MEDFORD** • PARRISH, EARL, M.D. • ROSS, DAVID A., M.D. **OREGON CITY** • HALE, LLOYD D., M.D. **PORTLAND** • ANDREWS, RICHARD P., M.D. • BIEKER, FRED W., M.D. • HAUGE, CHRISTOPHER W., M.D. • KANZLER, REINHOLD, M.D. • LINDGREN, VERNER V., M.D. • MARSHALL, WILLIAM R., M.D. • McCRAW, LOUIS H., JR., M.D. • MELVIN, MARCUS W., M.D. • MEYER, JAMES V., M.D. • PERRIN, EUGENE R., M.D. • SIMMONS, ROBERT D., M.D. • STARR, CHARLES R., M.D. • STEFFANOFF, DAN N., M.D. • STONE, ELIZABETH J., M.D. • TEN EYCK, JAMES R., M.D. • WEED, LINTON G., II, M.D. **SALEM** • GOTTSCHALK, WOLFRAM F., M.D.

PENNSYLVANIA

ALLENTOWN • ALTOBELLI, JOHN ANTHONY, M.D. • HEFFERNAN, ANDREW H., M.D. • MARCKS, KERWIN M., M.D. • OKUNSKI, WALTER J., M.D. • TREVASKIS, ALLEN E., M.D. **ALTOONA** • GIBBONS, WILLIAM P., M.D. **BETHLEHEM** • SALGADO, EDWARD M., M.D. **BRYN MAWR** • COLOMBO, JAMES L., M.D. • LAMP, J. CURTIS, M.D. • SOUSER, ROSYLN C., M.D. **CAMP HILL** • YATES, JAMES A., M.D. **CHADDS FORD** • DUNCAN, JOHN, M.D. **CHESTER** • OAKEY, RICHARD S., JR., M.D. **CHESTER SPRINGS** • BURGET, DEAN E., JR., M.D. **DANVILLE** • BROOKS, HAROLD W., M.D. **DOYLESTOWN** • HUNTER, MARVIN T., M.D. **ERIE** • BALES, CHARLES ROSS, M.D. • BAKER, GRAEME C., M.D. • TOOZE, FRANK M., M.D. **HARRISBURG** • HARDING, ROBERT L., M.D. • HERCEG, STEPHEN J., M.D. **HERSHEY** • DAVIS, THOMAS S., M.D. • GRAHAM, WILLIAM P., III, M.D. • MILLER, STEPHEN H., M.D. **JOHNSTOWN** • BENKO, STEPHEN T., M.D. **LANCASTER** • LONG, PHILIP M., M.D. **LEVITTOWN** • LAUANDOS, I. S., M.D. **NANTICOKE** • STARZYNSKI, T. E., M.D. **NORRISTOWN** • LUNDY, BARBARA S., M.D. **PHILADELPHIA** •

BROBYN, THOMAS J., M.D. • CHA, DONG S., M.D. • CHASE, ROBERT A., M.D. • CRAMER, LESTER M., M.D. • CULF, NORRIS K., M.D. • DAVIS, J. WALLACE, M.D. • HAMILTON, RALPH W., M.D. • HOLST, HAZEL I., M.D. • HULNICK, STUART J., M.D. • KODSI, MAGDI S., M.D. • LaROSSA, DONATO D., M.D. • LEHR, HERNDON BRIGGS, M.D. • MANSTEIN, GEORGE, M.D. • NOONE, R., BARRETT, M.D. • PRICE, RAPHAEL I. M., M.D. • RANDALL, PETER, M.D. • SCHEUERMANN, HENRY A., M.D. • SEITCHIK, MURRAY W., M.D. • SLAVIN, JAMES W., M.D. • THOROUGHGOOD, WILLIAM C., M.D. • WHITAKER, LINTON A., M.D. **PITTSBURGH** • ANDERSON, VICTOR S., M.D. • COHEN, BERNARD I., M.D. • CONKLIN, JAMES E., M.D. • GAISFORD, JOHN C., M.D. • GARRETT, WILLIAM S., JR., M.D. • HANNA, DWIGHT C., M.D. • MUSGRAVE, ROSS H., M.D. • NEFT, BURTON H., M.D. • RENTON, G. L., M.D. • RICHARDSON, GEORGE S., M.D. • SAMPSON, JOSEPH L., JR., M.D. • SKRENTA, RICHARD J., M.D. • VAGLEY, RICHARD T., M.D. • WHITE, WILLIAM L., M.D. • WORLEY, CARL M., M.D. **SCRANTON** • NAUSS, THOMAS J., M.D. **WEST READING** • MOSER, MANNY H., M.D. • PROSERPI, SERGIO V., M.D. **WILKES-BARRE** • CHUNG, CHAN KUN, M.D. **WILLIAMSPORT** • ECKER, HERBERT A., M.D. **YORK** • ANGELO, JOHN J., M.D. • DAVIS, ROBERT M., M.D.

RHODE ISLAND

PAWTUCKET • JEREMIAH, BERT S., M.D. • JOHNSON, CHARLES F., M.D. **PROVIDENCE** • SEXTON, RICHARD P., M.D. • STURIM, HOWARD S., M.D. • VERSACI, ARMAND D., M.D.

SOUTH CAROLINA

BEAUFORT • JENNINGS, HAL B., M.D. **CHARLESTON** • HAGERTY, ROBERT F., M.D. • HARVIN, J. SHAND, M.D. • MAGUIRE, CARTER P., M.D. • SCHUH, FREDRIC D., M.D. **COLUMBIA** • McLEAN, GEORGE E., M.D. **GREENVILLE** • ECKSTEIN, WILLIAM L., M.D. **HILTON HEAD ISLAND** • SMITH, J. ROY, M.D.

SOUTH DAKOTA

SIOUX FALLS • HUSSAIN, RIF'AT, M.D.

TENNESSEE

CHATTANOOGA • CRAFT, PHIL D., M.D. • DAVIS, JAMES WILSON, M.D. • HAYES, CAULEY W., JR., M.D. • LABRADOR, DANIEL, JR., M.D. • REYNOLDS, JOHN R., M.D. • RUSSELL, DONALD J., M.D. **JOHNSON CITY** • ARKEE, M. S. K., M.D. • CARVER, RICHARD F., M.D. **KNOXVILLE** • ANDREWS, EDMUND B., M.D. • COX, JAMES B., M.D. • HARPER, K. ALLEN, M.D. • KNOWLING, ROBERT E., M.D. **MEMPHIS** • ADAMS, LORENZO H., M.D. • ADAMS, WILLIAM MILTON, JR., M.D. • CLARENDON, COLIN C. D., M.D. • CRAVEN, RUFUS E., M.D. • DeMERE, McCARTHY, M.D. • HENDRIX, JAMES H., JR., M.D. • HUGHES, ALLEN H., M.D. • JEROME, ANTHONY P., M.D. • MURPHY, JAMES G., M.D. • REEDER, ROBERT C., M.D. • STEVENSON, ROBIN M., M.D. • VINCENT, JOHN ROBERT, M.D. • WALKER, JAMES W., M.D. • WHITE, CHARLES E., M.D. **NASHVILLE** • BOWERS, DAVID G., JR., M.D. • FLEMING, JAMES H., JR., M.D. • FRIST, JOHN C., M.D. • LYNCH, J. B., M.D. • MADDEN, JAMES J., JR., M.D. • ORCUTT, THOMAS W., M.D. • RICKETSON, GREER, M.D. • TODD, KIRKLAND W., JR., M.D.

TEXAS

ABILENE • WOLF, ROLAND O., M.D. **AMARILLO** • MOORE, JEFF R., M.D. **ARLINGTON** • DOYLE, JAMES E., M.D. • KORD, JOHN P., M.D. **AUSTIN** • BARNES, WILLIAM E., M.D. • BECKHAM, PATRICK H., M.D. • CLEMENT, ROBERT L., M.D. • MORRIS, FRANCIS A., JR., M.D. • PARKER, E. RICHARD, M.D. **BEAUMONT** • WASHBURN, W. W., JR., M.D. **BROWNSVILLE** • SOLEJA, KHLAID R., M.D. **CORPUS CHRISTI** • BALME, ROBERT H., M.D. • CONLEE, JACK LYNN, M.D. • GLANZ, SANFORD, M.D. **DALLAS** • ATKINS, RONALD W., M.D. • BARNES, RONALD E., M.D. • BARTON, FRITZ E., JR., M.D. • BLOOM, BERNARD H., M.D. • BROWN, BYRON LINSDAY, M.D. • CONNALLY, JOSEPH M., JR., M.D. • DEMUTH, ROBERT J., M.D. • DUNTON, EDWARD FRANK, M.D. • GASTON, ERSKIN A., M.D. • HAMRA, SAM T., M.D. • KIPP, DEAN C., M.D. • KLEIN, DONALD R., M.D. • LEMMON, MARK L., M.D. • LERMAN, MELVYN, M.D. • MELMED, EDWARD P., M.D. • NEWSOM, HAMLET T., M.D. • POLLOCK, HARLAN, M.D. • SALYER, KENNETH E., M.D. • SELLMAN, WILLARD C., M.D. • SMITH, SYDNIE G., M.D. **DENISON** • SWAMY, PONNUSWAMY T., M.D. **DENTON** • DYER, PEGGY J., M.D. **EL PASO** • BOGART, JOHN N., M.D. • EWALT, DONALD H., M.D. • GUM, RONALD A., M.D. • PANGMAN, W. JOHN, M.D. • PETERSON, JAMES F., M.D. • SCHUESSLER, W. W., M.D. • THERING, HARLAN R., M.D. **FORT SAM HOUSTON** • DUFFY, MICHAEL M., M.D. • NGAU, CURTIS A. M., M.D. • PETERSON, HUGH D., M.D. **FORT WORTH** • COERS, CARL R., III, M.D. • GRACIA, VALENTIN, M.D. • GRANT, DAVID ALAN, M.D. • HERR, DAVID R., M.D. • KHAN, SHUJAAT A., M.D. • PATTERSON, JOHN B., M.D. • TENERY, JOHN H., M.D. **FRIENDSWOOD** • HEMPHILL, JAMES E., M.D. **GALVESTON** • BLOCKER, TRUMAN G., JR., M.D. • HUANG, TED T., M.D. • LARSON, DUANE L., M.D. • LEWIS, STEPHEN R., M.D. • LOVE, H. G., JR., M.D. **HOUSTON** • ARFAI, PARVIZ, M.D. • BAILEY, CHARLES W., JR., M.D. • BARRETT, BERNARD M., JR., M.D. • BIGGS, THOMAS M., JR., M.D. • BOWEN, RALPH, M.D. • BRAUER, RAYMOND O., M.D. • CRAMER, ALAN T., M.D. • CRONIN, THOMAS D., M.D. • FREDERICKS, SIMON, M.D. • FREEMAN, BROMLEY S., M.D. • GARD, DON ALLAN, M.D. • GEROW, FRANK J., M.D. • HARDY, S. BARON, M.D. • KIRBY, EDWARD J., M.D. • MILLER, WILLIAM T., M.D. • MOORE, JAMES LEE, M.D. • OOI, SENG K., M.D. • REJAIE, IRAJ, M.D. • ROTHENBERG, PHILIP B., M.D. • SPIRA, MEL-VIN, M.D. • WIEMER, D. ROBERT, M.D. • WISE, ROBERT J., M.D. • WOLF, LAURENCE E., M.D. • WOOD, ROBERT W., JR., M.D. **LACKLAND AIR FORCE BASE** • BECKER, DAVID W., JR., M.D. • DENNIS, LeBARON W., M.D. • SHANKLIN, KENNETH D., M.D. **LUBBOCK** • KOCH, LEONARD, M.D. • ROWLEY, MILTON M., M.D. **McALLEN** • RIOS, LUIS MANUEL, M.D. **NACOGDOCHES** • GANNON, JOHN P., M.D. **PASADENA** • CANADA, WILLIAM

H., M.D. **PLANO** • TORANTO, I. RICHARD, M.D. **RICHARDSON** • CHANDLER, P. J., M.D. **SAN ANTONIO** • BALASUBRAMANIAN, R., M.D. • CARTER, JOHN E., M.D. • CROW, JUDSON L., M.D. • DOMINGUEZ, OSCAR J., M.D. • FORD, JOSEPH C., M.D. • GREER, DONALD M., M.D. • HOUSE, ROYCE E., M.D. • KNOX, JOHN STEPHEN, M.D. • SCHLATTNER, WILLIAM H., M.D. • SMITH, JAMES RALPH, M.D. • TENNISON, CHARLES W., M.D. • WILKINSON, TOLBERT S., M.D. **TEMPLE** • LYNCH, DENNIS J., M.D. • WHITE, RALEIGH R., IV, M.D. **TYLER** • BRELSFORD, H. GATES, M.D. • LeSAUVAGE, STEPHEN C., JR., M.D. **WEBSTER** • CHINOOKOSWONG, VRADEJ, M.D.

UTAH

OGDEN • BERGERA, JERALD J., M.D. • KEITER, JOHN E., M.D. • MALAN, LEE JEPPSON, M.D. **PROVO** • ROBERTSON, L. EUGENE, M.D. **SALT LAKE CITY** • BENSON, ARTHUR K., M.D. • BROADBENT, THOMAS RAY, M.D. • BROWNE, EARL Z., JR., M.D. • CLAYTON, JOHN L., M.D. • DINGMAN, DAVID L., M.D. • FAIRBANKS, GRANT R., M.D. • HICKMAN, GRANT A., M.D. • LEWIS, EDWARD C., II, M.D. • PICKENS, JAMES E., M.D. • ROBINSON, ROBERT R., JR., M.D. • SNYDER, CLIFFORD C., M.D. • WALKER, JAMES H., M.D. • WOOLF, ROBERT M., M.D. • YOUNGBLOOD, ROBERT L., M.D.

VERMONT

BURLINGTON • BARNEY, BERNARD B., M.D. • LINTON, PETER C., M.D.

VIRGINIA

ALEXANDRIA • McKNELLY, LAWRENCE O., M.D. **ARLINGTON** • AUSTIN, HARVEY, M.D. **CHARLOTTESVILLE** • EDGERTON, MILTON T., M.D. • FUTRELL, J. WILLIAM, M.D. • WILLIAMS, GAYLORD S., M.D. **FAIRFAX** • WHIPPLE, GEORGE A., M.D. **FALLS CHURCH** • ALEXANDER, JOHN E., M.D. • BLOCK, LEON I., M.D. • BORGES, ALBERT F., M.D. • CLIMO, MERRILL S., M.D. **McLEAN** • TEUNIS, BERNARD SCOTT, M.D. **NEWPORT NEWS** • LANIER, VERNE C., JR., M.D. • SHEPARD, GLENN H., M.D. **NORFOLK** • ADAMSON, JEROME E., M.D. CARRAWAY, JAMES H., M.D. • HORTON, CHARLES E., M.D. • McCRAW, JOHN B., M.D. • RUFFIN, WILLCOX, JR., M.D. • SHARZER, LEONARD A., M.D. **PORTSMOUTH** • MEEKINGS, WALTER J., JR., M.D. • SLEPYAN, DAVID H., M.D. • WALL, NORMAN R., M.D. **RICHMOND** • COHEN, I. KELMAN, M.D. • COLEMAN, CLAUDE C., JR., M.D. • JACKSON, HUNTER S., M.D. • MERRITT, WYNDELL H., M.D. • OLSHANSKY, KENNETH, M.D. • PETTY, CARROLL T., M.D. • ROWE, DOUGLAS S., M.D. • SMITH, LEROY, M.D. • THEOGARAJ, S. DAWSON, M.D. • WARE, J. LATANE, M.D. • WARTHEN, HARRY J., M.D. **ROANOKE** • BROBST, HENRY T., M.D. • KANG, YOUNG S., M.D. • MOORMAN, WARREN L., M.D. • MORRIS, JAMES C., III, M.D. • ROTH, ROBERT F., M.D. **ROSSLYN** • BELL, J. GORDON, M.D. **VIRGINIA BEACH** • MLADICK, RICHARD A., M.D. **WINCHESTER** • HIRSCHBERG, STANLEY M., M.D.

WASHINGTON

BELLEVUE • BERNER, CARL F., M.D. • LEFF, MICHAEL A., M.D. • MIDDLETON, A. GILMAN, M.D. **EDMONDS** • MILLER, JORDAN E., M.D. **EVERETT** • GOFORTH, VIRGIL A., M.D. **KIRKLAND** • NEU, BRUCE J., M.D. **OLYMPIA** • DICKASON, WAYNE L., M.D. • SMITH, SHERWOOD P., M.D. **SEATTLE** • BLUE, ALFRED I., M.D. • CHAMPION, WILLIAM M., M.D. • CHISM, CARL E., M.D. • DeVITO, ROBERT V., M.D. • EADE, GILBERT G., M.D. • KROPP, ROBERT J., M.D. • MOWERY, CHARLES S., M.D. • PILLING, MATTHEW A., M.D. • RICHEY, MACK D., M.D. • STURMAN, MELVIN J., M.D. • THORNE, FRANK L., M.D. • VASQUEZ, MARIO A., M.D. **SPOKANE** • BRINKMAN, JAMES F., M.D. • FOX, JOSEPH I., M.D. • JAMES, NORMAN J., M.D. • OLMSTED, GERALD W., M.D. • SULLIVAN, DAVID E., M.D. **TACOMA** • ALGER, JOHN R., M.D. • BANFIELD, ERNEST E., M.D. • BITSEFF, EDWARD L., M.D. • BRANDT, FRED A., M.D. • EKLAND, DAVID A., M.D. • IRISH, THOMAS J., JR., M.D. • STILWELL, JAMES R., M.D. • WHITE, HOBART J., M.D. **VANCOUVER** • BRAR, MANJIT I. S., M.D. **WENATCHEE** • TUCKER, KENNETH R., M.D. **YAKIMA** • KERR, WILSON J., M.D. • STILINOVIC, LAWRENCE M., M.D.

WEST VIRGINIA

CHARLESTON • CHARBONNIEZ, JACQUES, M.D. • LEE, HAN SEN, M.D. **HUNTINGTON** • GARMESTANI, ALI A., M.D. • HACKLEMAN, GENE L., M.D. **WHEELING** • McCONNELL, D. VERNE, M.D.

WISCONSIN

APPLETON • SCHINABECK, THOMAS J., M.D. **GREEN BAY** • JACOBS, EDMUND B., JR., M.D. **MADISON** • BERNARD, FRANK D., M.D. • DAVENPORT, GORDON, M.D. • DEMERGIAN, VAUGHN, M.D. • DIBBELL, DAVID G., M.D. • HAMACHER, JOHN EUGENE, M.D. **MARSHFIELD** • POUSTI, AHMED, M.D. **MILWAUKEE** • DAS, DILIP K., M.D. • DIX, C. ROBERT, M.D. • DOCKTOR, JOHN P., M.D. • ELIAS, SHARON L., M.D. • FRACKELTON, WILLIAM H., M.D. • GINGRASS, RUEDI P., M.D. • HOGAN, JOHN P., M.D. • HOWELL, ARTHUR, M.D. • KORKOS, GEORGE J., M.D. • KRETCHMAR, JOSEPH S., M.D. • LEVY, DONALD M., M.D. • NATVIG, PAUL, M.D. • POHL, ALAN L., M.D. • RIPPLE, HAROLD L., M.D. • TEASLEY, JACK LAMKIN, M.D. • WIVIOTT, WILBERT, M.D. • WYNN, SIDNEY K., M.D. **NEENAH** • SCHRANG, EUGENE A., M.D. **WATERTOWN** • PETERSON, FREDRICA N., M.D. **WAUWATOSA** • KLOEHN, RALPH A., M.D.

WYOMING

CHEYENNE • SLATER, PAUL V., M.D.

PUERTO RICO

GUAYNABO • SEGARRA, JOSE A., M.D. **HATO REY** • BENAVENT, WALTER J., M.D. **MAYAGUEZ** • RAMIREZ-IRIZARRY, ANGELA A., M.D. • VARGAS BUSQUETS, MIGUEL A., M.D. **SAN JUAN** • BARRETO, ARMANDO, M.D. • SANCHEZ, ALBERTO E., M.D.

AFRICA
ZAMBIA • SARGEANT, DONALD J., M.D.
COSTA RICA
SAN JOSE • MARTEN, ERNESTO, M.D.
INDIA
LUDHIANA • FEIRABEND, THEODORE C., M.D.
ICELAND
REYKJAVIK • THORVALDSSON, SIGURDUR EGILL, M.D.
IRAN
TEHRAN • FAIZ, MONOUCHER, M.D. • SAMIIAN, MOHAMAD REZA, M.D.
JORDAN
AMMAN • SHUBAILAT, GHAITH F., M.D.
LEBANON
BEIRUT • MAMOUN, SAMI M., M.D.
REPUBLIC OF SOUTH AFRICA
JOHANNESBURG • PENN, JOHN G., M.D. REPUBLIQUE DU ZAIRE • LEUZ, CHRISTOPHER A., III, M.D.
TAIWAN
TAIPEI • NOORDHOFF, M. SAMUEL, M.D.
THAILAND
BANGKOK • NILUBOL, PREEYAPHAS, M.D. • STHIENCHOAK, MANUS, M.D. • SUTHUNYARAT, PINIT, M.D. HAEDYAI • PREMASATHIAN, DILOK, M.D.
VENEZUELA
CARACUS • MONDOLFI, PAUL E., M.D.
DOMINION OF CANADA
ALBERTA
EDMONTON • VOLOSHIN, PETER J., M.D.
BRITISH COLUMBIA
NEW WESTMINSTER • RAI, DYALCHAND KIMIT, M.D.
MANITOBA
WINNIPEG • SNELLING, CHARLES F. T., M.D.
NEW BRUNSWICK
MONCTON • INGLIS, DOUGLAS S., M.D.
ONTARIO
HAMILTON • HEDDLE, STEWART B., M.D. LONDON • HURST, LAWRENCE N., M.D. TORONTO • FARMER, ALFRED W., M.D. • GORDON, STUART D., M.D. • LINDSAY, WILLIAM K., M.D. • MUNRO, IAN ROSS, M.D.
QUEBEC
MONTREAL • BAXTER, HAMILTON, M.D. • COHEN, JACK, M.D. • DANIEL, ROLLIN K., M.D. • ENTIN, MARTIN A., M.D. • PERRAS, COLETTE, M.D. • WILLIAMS, H. BRUCE, M.D. PIEDMONT • GERRIE, JOHN W., M.D. ST. HYACINTHE • CHARBONNEAU, IVAN, M.D.
GRANTED FOREIGN CERTIFICATION
ABU-JAMRA, FAWZI N., M.D. • ANTYPAS, PHILIP G., M.D. • ARREGUI, JAIME ALBA, M.D. • AU, OTTO YUM-TO, M.D. • BANUELOS, JOSE A. RODA, M.D. • BHOKAKUL, PRATEEP, M.D. • BIN, JOO WON, M.D. • BINDRA, RAVINDER NATH, M.D. • BOSKOVIC, DARINKA M., M.D. • CALOSTYPIS, FANNY, M.D. • CALZOLARI, LEANDRO, M.D. • CHAROONSMITH, THAVORN, M.D. • CHUNEKAMRAI, DISPONG, M.D. • CLODIUS, LEANDRO, M.D. • COLE, OWEN RUSSELL, M.D. • DUPIUS, CHRISTIAN C., M.D. • DUR-RANI, KHALID M. H., M.D. • ESPALDON, ERNESTO M., M.D. • FUJINO, TOYOMI, M.D. • GARCIA-VELASCO, JOSE, M.D. • GHAVAMI, MOHSEN POUR, M.D. • GLIOSCI, AMLETO, M.D. • HIRAYAMA, TAKESHI, M.D. • HITA, JOSE CASTILLO, M.D. • JAMAL, SINNAMO-HIDEEN, M.D. • KANDIAH, SIVANANTHARAJ, M.D. • KOEHNLEIN, M. EDZARD, M.D. • KOLLIOPOULOS, PANAGIOTIS K., M.D. • LEW, JAE DUK, M.D. • MANI, MANI M., M.D. • MARGARIDE, LUIS ALBERTO, M.D. • MATTON, GUIDO, M.D. • MONTANDON, DENYS, M.D. • OGO, KEN, M.D. • PANDYA, NARENDRA J., M.D. • PASHA, M. NAJDAT IBRAHIM, M.D. • PATEL, MAHENDRAKUMAR P., M.D. • PEETERS, RUDOLF LEO, M.D. • PUNYA-HOTRA, VICHIT, M.D. • REMON, JOSE A., M.D. • REYSIO-CRUZ, MARCELINO, JR., M.D. • RUBEIZ, MICHEL TANIOS, M.D. • SHEHADI, SAMEER I., M.D. • SHERKAT, MEHDI, M.D. • SHIOYA, NOBUYUKI, M.D. • SRIVASTAVA, DINESH C., M.D. • SUDACHIT, PRASARN, M.D. • TSUR, HAGGAI, M.D. • ULLAO-GREGORI, A. OSCAR, M.D. • VANDE-PUT, JACQUES, M.D. • VELUPILLAI, SIVALOGANATHAN, M.D. • VILLORIA, JOSE M. FERNANDEZ, M.D. • VREBOS, JACQUES E. R., M.D. • YAGHNAM, FARID CONSTANDI, M.D.

INDEX

NOTE: Italic page numbers indicate illustrations.

Riding breeches deformity
anesthesia for, 127
procedure, 127-129
scarring from, 128-129

Scarring
from abdominoplasty, 120, *121*
from breast lift surgery, 99
from breast reduction surgery,
104, 105
from hip and thigh surgery,
126, 128-129
Schadow, 54
Silastic, 85
Silicone gel, 85
Skin
biochemical changes in, 5
blood flow to, 5
excess above elbow, 131
hanging, on arm, 131-133
sagging, 4-6
and smoking, 5
types, 13, 31
and weight loss, 5
Skin tone, loss of, 5
Sleep, effects on skin, 5-6

Smell, loss of, due to nasal
surgery, 66
Smoking, effects on skin circu-
lation, 5
Strombeck, 103
Sun blocking agents, 21, 30
Sunlight, postoperative exposure
to, 20-21, 30, 63
Swelling, after surgery, 19, 23,
29, 34, 59, 63

Tears
excessive from eyelid surgery,
41
lack of, from eyelid surgery,
41-42
Temporal area (face)
extent of, 4, 6-7
operation on, 7
problems in, 7
Thrombophlebitis. *See* Blood clots
Thymol iodide powder, 29
"Turkey gobbler" appearance,
correction of, 9-10

Valium®, 38
Virginal breast hypertrophy, 102

166